Chia Seeds for Constipation in Kids

Happy Tummies, Happy Kids! Unlock the Power of Chia Seeds for Natural Relief

Alice Klayn

DISCLAIMER 5

INTRODUCTION 6

CHAPTER 1: UNDERSTANDING CONSTIPATION IN KIDS.............. 8

Causes of Constipation in Children 11
Symptoms and Diagnosis of Constipation in Children 15

CHAPTER 2: THE NUTRITIONAL POWER OF CHIA SEEDS 20

How Chia Seeds Can Help Constipation in Children 24
Nutritional Profile and Benefits of chia seeds 28

CHAPTER 3: HOW CHIA SEEDS AID DIGESTION 33

Fiber Content and Its Role chia seeds 36
Hydration and Gel Formation in chia seeds 39

CHAPTER 4: INTRODUCING CHIA SEEDS TO YOUR CHILD'S DIET.. 44

Safe Dosages and Recommendations When Using Chia Seeds for Children 47
Creative Ways to Include Chia Seeds for Kids............................ 50

CHAPTER 5: TASTY CHIA SEED RECIPES FOR KIDS 56

Breakfast Boosters including Chia Seeds for Kids 60
Snack Time Favorites Including Chia Seeds for Kids 65

CHAPTER 6: HYDRATION AND ITS IMPORTANCE FOR CONSTIPATION 70

Why Kids Need Plenty of Water 74
Chia Seeds and Hydration... 77

CHAPTER 7: MONITORING YOUR CHILD'S PROGRESS WHEN CONSUMING CHIA SEEDS.. 81

Keeping a Food Diary when consuming chia seeds............................ 84
Identifying Improvement when consuming chia seeds 88

CHAPTER 8: ADDRESSING COMMON CONCERNS WHEN INCLUDING CHIA SEEDS IN CHILDREN'S DIETS........................ 93

Allergies and Intolerances in Children 96
Potential Side Effects of Using Chia Seeds in Children's Diets 99

CHAPTER 9: ADDITIONAL NATURAL REMEDIES FOR

CONSTIPATION IN CHILDREN..102

Complementary Foods and Practices for Constipation in Children 107
Lifestyle Changes for Better Digestion for Constipation in Children 111

CHAPTER 10: CHIA SEEDS BEYOND CONSTIPATION....................115

Other Health Benefits of Chia Seeds for Kids...118
Long-term Dietary Inclusion of Chia Seeds for Children 121

CONCLUSION...125

BIOGRAPHY 126

BONUS 01: CHIA-SEED-HEALTH-TRACKER-FOR-KIDS................128

BONUS 02: CHIA-SEED-RECIPE-FOR-CONSTIPATION-IN-KIDS
....128

BONUS 03: CHIA-SEEDS-CREATIVE-MEAL-PLANNING-FOR-KIDS 128

GLOSSARY: CHIA SEEDS FOR CONSTIPATION KIDS....................129

Disclaimer

The information provided in this book, "Chia Seeds for Constipation Kids: Happy Tummies, Happy Kids! Unlock the Power of Chia Seeds for Natural Relief," by Alice Klayn, is intended solely for educational purposes. It is designed to offer general information and insights into the use of chia seeds for addressing constipation in children.

Always seek the advice of your physician or other qualified healthcare provider with any questions you may have regarding a medical condition. Never disregard professional medical advice or delay in seeking it because of something you have read in this book.

Introduction

Welcome to **"Chia Seeds for Constipation: A Parent's Guide to Natural Relief for Kids,"** where the journey to your child's digestive health begins. I'm Alice Klayn, a dedicated expert in nutrition and digestive health with over a decade of experience transforming lives through holistic wellness. My passion for understanding the human gut and my mission to find natural, effective remedies for common digestive issues have led me to uncover the incredible benefits of chia seeds.

As a parent, watching your child struggle with constipation can be heart-wrenching. The discomfort, the tears, and the endless search for a solution can leave you feeling helpless.

 But what if I told you there's a simple, natural way to bring relief and restore your child's digestive health? This book is designed to guide you through the wonders of chia seeds—a tiny superfood packed with fiber, nutrients, and gut-healing properties.

Understand how these tiny seeds work their magic in promoting regular bowel movements and overall gut health.

Delightful and easy-to-make recipes that incorporate chia seeds into your child's diet, making mealtime both nutritious and enjoyable.

Expert advice on incorporating chia seeds into everyday meals, ensuring your child gets the full benefits without any fuss.

Inspiring accounts from parents who have witnessed the transformative effects of chia seeds on their children's digestive health.

This book is more than just a guide—it's a lifeline for parents seeking natural, effective solutions to help their children overcome constipation. With my warm, approachable style and unwavering commitment to health, I'm here to support you every step of the way. Together, let's embark on this transformative journey towards a healthier, happier life for your child.

Chapter 1: Understanding Constipation in Kids

Constipation is a common issue that many children face at some point in their development. Understanding the complexities of this condition is essential for parents, caregivers, and educators, as it can significantly affect a child's well-being, behavior, and overall quality of life. In this chapter, we will explore the definition of constipation, its prevalence in children, contributing factors, and associated symptoms and complications.

What is Constipation?

Constipation is generally defined as infrequent bowel movements or difficulty passing stools that persist over a period of time. While bowel habits can vary widely from one child to another, most experts agree that a child is considered constipated when they have fewer than three bowel movements per week, experience painful bowel movements, or have hard, dry stools.

In children, constipation can be acute (short-term) or chronic (long-term), with chronic constipation being a condition that can last for several months or years. It is important to understand that occasional episodes of constipation are common among children, but they can become a recurrent problem that needs attention and intervention.

Prevalence of Constipation in Children

Studies suggest that constipation affects approximately 3% to 25% of the pediatric population, with variations depending on factors such as age, gender, and dietary habits. Infants are less likely to experience constipation;

however, as children transition to solid foods (usually between 6 months and one year), the incidence begins to increase. The early childhood and preschool years are particularly critical as children start to exercise independence over their food choices and bathroom habits.

It is also important to note that constipation appears to be more common in boys than in girls, particularly in the early years of life, although this trend may even out as children grow older. Regardless of gender, psychological aspects (such as fears of using the bathroom or changes in routine) can play a significant role in a child's gut health.

Causes of Constipation

A variety of factors can contribute to constipation in children, including:

Dietary Factors: A diet low in fiber, which is found in fruits, vegetables, and whole grains, can lead to hard stools. The absence of adequate fluids may also exacerbate the problem, as hydration is essential for maintaining soft stool consistency.

Inactivity: Children who lead a sedentary lifestyle may find it more challenging to have regular bowel movements. Physical activity stimulates bowel movements, and a lack of exercise can slow down digestion.

Toilet Training: The process of toilet training can be a stressful experience for some children, leading to anxiety around using the toilet. This anxiety may result in withholding stools, which can aggravate constipation.

Psychological Factors: Emotional stressors, such as

changes in routine (moving to a new home, starting school, or family disruptions), can impact a child's bowel habits. Fear of pain associated with bowel movements can lead to avoidance behavior, creating a cycle that perpetuates constipation.

Medical Conditions: In some cases, underlying medical conditions—such as hypothyroidism, neurological disorders, or gastrointestinal malformations—may result in constipation. Children who are on certain medications that have constipation as a side effect may also face difficulties.

Symptoms of Constipation

Recognizing the symptoms of constipation can help parents take appropriate action. Common symptoms include:

Infrequent bowel movements (less than three times per week)

Difficulty or discomfort while passing stools

Hard, dry, or pellet-like stools

Abdominal pain or cramping

A feeling of incomplete evacuation after a bowel movement

Bloating

Irritability or behavioral changes in younger children ## Complications of Constipation

If left unaddressed, constipation can lead to various complications. Children may experience fecal impaction, where a large mass of stool becomes stuck in the rectum, causing pain and potentially leading to further issues. This can result in the child becoming emotionally distressed or embarrassed, leading to a worsening cycle of withholding stools.

Additionally, chronic constipation may affect a child's appetite and lead to dietary issues or malnutrition. Over time, constipation can also impact a child's social interactions and confidence, particularly if they're reluctant to use bathrooms outside their home environment.

As we move forward in this book, we will delve deeper into strategies for prevention, management, and lifestyle changes that can help alleviate this common yet often misunderstood condition. Through education and open dialogue, we can help our children lead healthier, happier lives free from the discomfort associated with constipation.

Causes of Constipation in Children

It can be distressing not only for the child but also for parents and caregivers who want to see their children healthy and comfortable. Understanding the causes of constipation in children is crucial for effective prevention and management. This chapter will explore the various factors contributing to constipation, ranging from dietary choices to psychological influences.

1. Dietary Factors

a. Insufficient Fiber Intake

One of the primary causes of constipation in children is a diet low in fiber. Fiber aids digestion and adds bulk to stools, making them easier to pass. Many children consume diets high in processed foods and low in fruits, vegetables, and whole grains, which can lead to inadequate fiber intake. Increasing the consumption of fiber-rich foods, such as apples, pears, carrots, and whole grains, can help provide the necessary nutrients that promote regular bowel movements.

b. Dehydration

Hydration plays a critical role in maintaining healthy bowel function. When children do not drink enough fluids, their bodies absorb more water from the food in the intestines, leading to harder, drier stools that are difficult to pass. Parents should encourage children to drink plenty of water throughout the day, especially when they are active, to prevent dehydration-related constipation.

2. Physical Factors ### a. Sedentary Lifestyle

A lack of physical activity can contribute to constipation in children. Sedentary behaviors, such as excessive screen time, can slow down the digestive system, making bowel movements less frequent. Encouraging regular physical activity, such as outdoor play, sports, or family walks, can stimulate digestion and help maintain regular bowel habits.

b. Medical Conditions

Certain medical conditions can also lead to constipation. Conditions such as hypothyroidism, neurological disorders, and gastrointestinal abnormalities can affect the motility of the digestive system. Children with these conditions may require medical evaluation and treatment to manage their constipation effectively.

Parents should consult healthcare professionals if they suspect an underlying medical issue. ## 3. Psychological Factors

a. Anxiety and Stress

Emotional factors can significantly influence a child's bowel habits. Anxiety, stress, and changes in routine—such as starting school, family relocation, or parental divorce—can lead to constipation. Children may develop a fear of using the toilet, especially if they experience pain during bowel movements. This can create a negative feedback loop where the child avoids going to the bathroom, ultimately leading to further constipation. Addressing emotional well-being and fostering a positive environment around toilet habits is crucial for helping children overcome psychological barriers.

b. Toilet Training and Habits

The process of toilet training can also impact a child's bowel habits. Some children may resist using the toilet, preferring the comfort of a diaper. Additionally, if a child is regularly forced to hold in their stool while waiting for a convenient time to use the bathroom, this can lead to constipation. Establishing a regular toilet routine, offering praise for successes, and addressing any fears associated with using the toilet can help prevent constipation during this transitional phase.

4. Medications

Certain medications can have constipation as a side effect. For example, over-the-counter pain relievers, some antacids, and iron supplements may cause or worsen constipation. If a child is experiencing constipation and is taking medication, it is essential for parents to consult with a healthcare provider.

Adjusting the medication or supplement dosage or considering alternatives may help alleviate the issue. ## 5. Environmental Factors

a. School and Social Settings

Children often face changes in their environment, particularly when transitioning to school. Factors such as unfamiliar toilets, time constraints during bathroom breaks, or peer pressure to avoid using public restrooms can lead children to postpone bowel movements, resulting in constipation. Educating children about the importance of listening to their bodies and going to the bathroom when they feel the urge can help foster healthier habits.

b. Travel

Traveling can disrupt a child's normal routine, including their eating and bathroom habits. Changes in diet, schedule, and lack of familiar bathroom facilities can contribute to constipation. Parents can prepare for travel by ensuring their children have access to fiber-rich snacks and maintaining regular hydration.

In conclusion, constipation in children can arise from a myriad of causes, including dietary choices, physical activity levels, psychological factors, medication use, and environmental influences. Awareness of these causes allows parents and caregivers to proactively address the issue and implement strategies to promote healthy bowel habits.

Symptoms and Diagnosis of Constipation in Children

It encompasses more than just infrequent bowel movements; it entails a variety of symptoms that can significantly affect a child's well-being and quality of life. This chapter aims to elucidate the symptoms associated with constipation in children, as well as to provide a systematic approach to diagnosis.

Definition of Constipation

Constipation is generally defined as having fewer than three bowel movements per week. However, in children, this definition must be contextualized, as normal bowel patterns can vary widely based on factors such as age, diet, and level of physical activity. It is crucial to consider the child's individual baseline when discussing constipation.

Symptoms of Constipation

Infrequent Bowel Movements:

Many parents first suspect constipation when children go more than two or three days without having a bowel movement. It's important to note that frequency alone does not determine constipation.

Hard, Dry Stools:

Children with constipation often have stools that are hard, dry, and difficult to pass. This can lead to pain, causing children to avoid subsequent bowel movements altogether.

Abdominal Pain or Discomfort:

Some children may experience cramping or discomfort in their abdomen. They may verbally express their discomfort or show signs of distress.

Straining During Bowel Movements:

Observing a child straining, grimacing, or taking a long time in the bathroom can indicate that they are struggling to pass stool. Frequent prolonged periods in the bathroom can raise concern.

Fecal Soiling (Encopresis):

A child may pass small amounts of stool unintentionally, which can often be mistaken for diarrhea. This can happen when a large, impacted stool obstructs the rectum, leading to leakage.

Loss of Appetite:

Some children may eat less or show a decreased interest in food due to discomfort or pain associated with their bowel movements.

Behavioral Changes:

Constipation can lead to behavioral issues such as irritability, anxiety around toilet use, and changes in mood. Children may become resistant to using the toilet out of fear of pain.

Family History:

Parents may notice patterns of constipation within the family, highlighting genetic or environmental factors contributing to the issue.

Diagnosing Constipation

The diagnosis of constipation in children involves a thorough clinical assessment, which includes:

1. Medical History

Gathering Information: A healthcare provider often begins by taking a detailed medical history. This includes questions about the child's dietary habits, frequency and consistency of bowel movements, fluid intake, and any episodes of pain or discomfort.

Developmental Factors: Assessing the child's developmental milestones, toilet training status, and any recent stressors or changes in routine (like starting school) is also crucial.

2. Physical Examination

Abdominal Examination: A careful examination of the abdomen can reveal signs of stool impaction or discomfort. The provider may palpate for distension or masses.

Rectal Examination: In some cases, a rectal examination may be performed to assess for impactation or other rectal abnormalities. While this may be uncomfortable for the child, it is essential for an accurate diagnosis.

3. Observing Bowel Patterns

Bowel Diary: Parents may be asked to keep a bowel diary for a specific period, noting the frequency and consistency of bowel movements. This can provide valuable insights for healthcare providers.

4. Laboratory Tests

When Necessary: Routine laboratory tests are

generally not required for diagnosing typical constipation. However, in cases where there are concerns regarding an underlying disease (such as endocrine disorders), blood tests or imaging studies may be recommended.

5. Differential Diagnosis

Exclusion of Other Conditions: It is vital to differentiate functional constipation from secondary causes such as metabolic disorders, structural abnormalities, or gastrointestinal diseases. Understanding the context and duration of symptoms is crucial in establishing whether constipation is primary (functional) or secondary.

6. Referral to a Specialist

Pediatric Gastroenterology: In complex cases or when initial treatments fail to yield improvements, referring the child to a pediatric gastroenterologist may be necessary for further evaluation and management.

Identifying and understanding the symptoms of constipation in children is essential in providing timely and appropriate interventions. Diagnosing constipation requires a multifaceted approach, considering both clinical history and physical examination, to ensure accurate conclusions are drawn for effective management.

Chapter 2: The Nutritional Power of Chia Seeds

Derived from the Salvia hispanica plant, these tiny seeds—often no bigger than a pinhead—pack a remarkable nutritional punch. Once a staple in ancient diets of the Aztecs and Mayans, chia seeds have resurfaced in modern health consciousness as a superfood, prized for their versatility and nutritional profile. In this chapter, we will explore the myriad benefits of chia seeds, their composition, and how incorporating them into our diets can enhance overall health and well-being.

1. Nutritional Composition

To fully appreciate the power of chia seeds, one must first examine their composition. A single ounce (about two tablespoons) of chia seeds contains approximately:

Calories: 138

Protein: 4.7 grams

Fat: 8.6 grams (of which 5 grams are omega-3 fatty acids)

Carbohydrates: 12 grams

Fiber: 10.6 grams

Calcium: 18% of the Recommended Daily Allowance (RDA)

Manganese: 30% of the RDA

Magnesium: 24% of the RDA

Phosphorus: 27% of the RDA

Zinc: 12% of the RDA

Antioxidants: Various forms, including quercetin, kaempferol, and chlorogenic acid

The most striking characteristic of chia seeds is their high omega-3 fatty acid content, particularly alpha- linolenic acid (ALA), which plays a crucial role in heart health and inflammation reduction. Alongside omega-3s, their impressive fiber content contributes to gut health and feelings of satiety.

1.1 Omega-3 Fatty Acids: The Heart's Best Friend

Omega-3 fatty acids, often lauded for their cardiovascular benefits, are essential fats that the body cannot produce on its own. Consuming chia seeds regularly can help improve heart health by lowering blood pressure and cholesterol levels, and reducing the risk of heart disease. Moreover, omega-3 fatty acids are known to support brain function and may even mitigate symptoms of depression and anxiety.

1.2 Fiber: Fuel for the Gut

Chia seeds are one of the richest plant sources of fiber. Their soluble fiber content swells when mixed with water, forming a gel-like substance that aids in digestion. This property not only helps regulate bowel movements but also supports a healthy gut microbiome, vital for nutrient absorption and overall digestive health. Additionally, the fiber in chia seeds can contribute to weight management by promoting a feeling of fullness.

1.3 Antioxidants: The Body's Protectors

Chia seeds are also abundant in antioxidants, compounds that combat oxidative stress caused by free radicals in the body. This protective quality may reduce the risk of chronic diseases, including cancer and heart disease. By neutralizing harmful substances, antioxidants play a pivotal role in preserving cellular health and may enhance longevity.

2. Health Benefits

With such a remarkable nutritional profile, it is no surprise that chia seeds offer a plethora of health benefits.
2.1 Weight Management

One of the most sought-after benefits of chia seeds is their potential to aid in weight loss. Their high fiber content slows digestion, promoting prolonged feelings of fullness. This can help individuals consume fewer calories throughout the day while still feeling satisfied. Moreover, chia seeds can be easily added to various meals and snacks, making them a convenient addition to weight management strategies.

2.2 Bone Health

Chia seeds are rich in calcium, magnesium, and phosphorus—all of which are vital for maintaining strong bones. Incorporating chia seeds into one's diet may help prevent osteoporosis and promote bone density, especially in populations at risk, such as postmenopausal women.

2.3 Heart Health

Numerous studies underscore the heart-health benefits of chia seeds. Their ability to lower blood pressure, reduce inflammation, and improve lipid profiles positions them as a heart-friendly food. Regular consumption of chia seeds can be an integral part of a heart-healthy diet.

2.4 Diabetes Control

Emerging evidence suggests that chia seeds may help regulate blood sugar levels, making them particularly beneficial for those with diabetes. The soluble fiber and healthy fats in chia seeds can slow glucose absorption and improve insulin sensitivity, ultimately aiding in blood sugar management.

3. Culinary Versatility

One of the most appealing aspects of chia seeds is their culinary versatility. They have a mild, nutty flavor that allows them to be easily incorporated into various dishes. Whether sprinkled over salads, blended into smoothies, or used as an egg substitute in baking, chia seeds can enhance the nutritional quality of your meals without altering their taste.

3.1 Chia Pudding

One of the simplest and most popular ways to enjoy chia seeds is through chia pudding. By soaking chia seeds in milk (dairy or non-dairy) or yogurt overnight, you create a creamy, nutrient-packed treat that can be customized with fruits, nuts, and sweeteners to suit your palate.

3.2 Smoothies

Adding chia seeds to smoothies not only thickens the texture but also boosts the nutrient content. Their slimy consistency, when soaked, can also make your smoothie more filling, providing sustained energy throughout the day.

3.3 Baking

Chia seeds can be used as a binding agent in baking. Combined with water, they form a gel that mimics the texture of eggs, making them a popular choice for vegan recipes.

As we have explored in this chapter, chia seeds are truly a nutritional powerhouse. Their rich profile of healthy fats, fiber, protein, vitamins, and minerals make them a valuable addition to any diet. The health benefits ranging from improved heart health to enhanced digestive function underscore their status as a superfood. By incorporating chia seeds into our daily routines, we can harness their potential to promote

better health and lead enriched lives.

How Chia Seeds Can Help Constipation in Children

As parents and caregivers seek effective and gentle remedies, chia seeds have gained popularity for their potential health benefits, particularly for digestive health. This chapter delves into the properties of chia seeds, how they can alleviate constipation in children, and practical ways to incorporate them into your child's diet.

Understanding Constipation in Children

Constipation is defined as infrequent bowel movements, typically fewer than three times a week, accompanied by hard, difficult-to-pass stools. In children, constipation can be caused by various factors, including inadequate fluid intake, low fiber diets, lack of physical activity, and stress. It can also be the result of withholding bowel movements due to fear or discomfort.

Signs and Symptoms

Parents should be aware of the following signs that may indicate constipation in their child:

Infrequent bowel movements

Hard or dry stools

Painful defecation

Abdominal pain or discomfort

Bloating or excessive gas

Reduced appetite or reluctance to eat ## The Nutritional Power of Chia Seeds

Chia seeds are tiny black seeds derived from the Salvia hispanica plant, native to Central and South America. They are rich in essential nutrients that contribute to overall health, making them a valuable addition to a child's diet:

High in Fiber: Chia seeds are an excellent source of soluble and insoluble fiber. For children, fiber is crucial for maintaining healthy digestion and preventing constipation.

Omega-3 Fatty Acids: These healthy fats are important for brain development and overall health. While not directly linked to constipation relief, they support overall bodily functions.

Hydration: Chia seeds can absorb up to 12 times their weight in water, forming a gel-like substance. This property can help to keep the digestive tract well-hydrated and promote softer stools.

Rich in Antioxidants: Antioxidants in chia seeds can

help combat inflammation and support overall digestive health.

How Chia Seeds Alleviate Constipation

The combination of high fiber content and the unique gel-forming capacity of chia seeds makes them a natural remedy for constipation. When chia seeds are consumed, they swell and create a gel-like substance in the stomach. This gel not only aids in stool passage but also promotes regular bowel movements.

Mechanisms at Work

Increased Fiber Intake: The soluble fiber in chia seeds helps to add bulk to the stool, making it easier to pass. It also regulates the speed at which food moves through the digestive tract.

Hydration: As chia seeds absorb water, they provide a hydrating effect that can help soften stools, making them easier to eliminate.

Prebiotic Properties: The fiber in chia seeds acts as a prebiotic, feeding the good bacteria in the gut. A healthy gut microbiome is crucial for effective digestion and regular bowel movements.

Incorporating Chia Seeds into Your Child's Diet

Introducing chia seeds to your child's diet can be both easy and fun. Here are several creative ways to incorporate them:

Chia Seed Pudding: Mix chia seeds with milk (dairy or plant-based) and a sweetener like honey or maple syrup. Allow the mixture to sit overnight in the refrigerator for a tasty and nutritious dessert or breakfast.

Smoothies: Add a tablespoon of chia seeds to your child's favorite smoothie. The seeds will blend in without altering the flavor while providing added nutrition.

Baked Goods: Substitute a portion of flour with ground chia seeds in recipes for pancakes, muffins, or bread. This not only boosts fiber content but also adds omega-3 fatty acids.

Yogurt Toppings: Sprinkle chia seeds on top of yogurt with fruits and nuts for a healthy snack.

Soups and Stews: Stir chia seeds into soups or stews to thicken the broth while adding nutritional benefits.

Important Considerations

While chia seeds are generally safe for children, it's important to follow a few precautions:

Start Small: Introduce chia seeds gradually. A teaspoon a day is a good starting point for younger children. Monitor for any digestive changes and adjust the quantity as necessary.

Hydration: Ensure your child drinks enough fluids throughout the day, as fiber works best when combined with adequate hydration.

Observe Reactions: Keep an eye on how your child responds to chia seeds. If any adverse reactions occur, consult a pediatrician.

By incorporating chia seeds into your child's meals in fun and creative ways, you can help ensure they remain comfortable, healthy, and happy. As with any dietary change, it's best to consult with a healthcare professional to tailor approaches that suit your child's specific needs.

With a little creativity and care, chia seeds can become a valuable ally in your child's journey towards better digestive health.

Nutritional Profile and Benefits of chia seeds

Originating from the Salvia hispanica plant, which is native to Mexico and Guatemala, these tiny, nutrient-dense seeds have been a staple in the diets of ancient civilizations such as the Aztecs and Mayans for centuries. In this chapter, we will explore the comprehensive nutritional profile of chia seeds, their myriad health benefits, and practical ways to incorporate them into our diets.

Nutritional Profile of Chia Seeds

Chia seeds are remarkably small yet boast an impressive array of nutrients. A typical serving size is about 28 grams (approximately two tablespoons), which contains:

Calories: 138

Protein: 4.7 grams

Fat: 8.6 grams (mostly polyunsaturated fats, including omega-3 fatty acids)

Carbohydrates: 12 grams

Fiber: 10.6 grams

Calcium: 177 mg

Magnesium: 95 mg

Phosphorus: 244 mg

Potassium: 116 mg

Iron: 1 mg

Zinc: 1 mg

Antioxidants: Various phenolic compounds are present.

Chia seeds are particularly high in omega-3 fatty acids, specifically alpha-linolenic acid (ALA), which is crucial for heart and brain health. They are also rich in dietary fiber, which contributes to digestive health and promotes satiety.

Another notable aspect of chia seeds is their unique ability to absorb water. When soaked, they can swell to up to 10-12 times their weight, forming a gel-like substance. This property not only enhances their versatility in recipes but also aids in hydration and prolonging feelings of fullness.

Health Benefits of Chia Seeds ### 1. Heart Health

The high omega-3 fatty acid content in chia seeds contributes to cardiovascular health by reducing inflammation, decreasing blood pressure, and lowering cholesterol levels. Regular consumption of chia seeds has been associated with reduced risk factors for heart disease, thus supporting overall heart health and functioning.

2. Digestive Health

The abundant dietary fiber found in chia seeds promotes regular bowel movements and supports digestive health. The soluble fiber helps in maintaining gut flora, while the gel-like consistency aids in smooth transit through the digestive tract. Incorporating chia seeds into meals can alleviate constipation and contribute to overall gut health.

3. Weight Management

Chia seeds can be a valuable ally in weight management. Their high fiber content promotes feelings of fullness, helping to curb appetite and reduce overall calorie intake. When consumed before meals, chia seeds can expand in the stomach, leading to prolonged satiety and less frequent snacking.

4. Bone Health

Rich in calcium, magnesium, and phosphorus, chia seeds are an excellent addition to a diet aimed at improving bone health. These minerals play a crucial role in maintaining bone density and strength, making chia seeds a beneficial choice for individuals seeking to support their skeletal system, especially in the absence of dairy.

5. Blood Sugar Regulation

The fiber content in chia seeds slows down the absorption of sugar, which can help stabilize blood sugar levels. This is particularly beneficial for individuals with diabetes or those at risk of developing the condition. Incorporating chia seeds into meals can promote a more gradual release of glucose into the bloodstream, thus minimizing spikes and crashes.

6. Antioxidant Properties

Chia seeds are packed with antioxidants, which play a vital role in combating oxidative stress and reducing inflammation in the body. These compounds can help prevent cellular damage, lower the risk of chronic diseases, and promote overall health and longevity.

7. Versatility and Easy Incorporation

Chia seeds can be easily integrated into a variety of dishes, making them a convenient health-enhancing addition to any diet. They can be sprinkled on salads, blended into smoothies, added to yogurt, or used in baking recipes. Due to their neutral flavor, they complement both sweet and savory dishes seamlessly.

Whether one is looking to improve heart health, promote digestive wellness, manage weight, strengthen bones, regulate blood sugar levels, or simply explore new nutritious foods, chia seeds offer an accessible and versatile solution. As we move forward in our quest for optimal health and wellness, these tiny seeds can be a cornerstone of a balanced and nourishing diet, empowering us to harness their full potential.

Chapter 3: How Chia Seeds Aid Digestion

Primarily recognized for their high nutritional value, these tiny seeds boast an impressive composition of omega-3 fatty acids, fiber, protein, vitamins, and minerals. One of the most compelling areas of research surrounding chia seeds is their impact on digestive health. In this chapter, we will explore the numerous ways chia seeds aid digestion by examining their fiber content, unique properties, and practical applications.

The Fiber Factor

One of the most notable characteristics of chia seeds is their high fiber content. In just one ounce (approximately 28 grams) of chia seeds, you can find about 10 grams of dietary fiber. This combination of soluble and insoluble fiber is what makes chia seeds particularly beneficial for digestion.

Soluble Fiber: A Gelatinous Marvel

When mixed with liquid, chia seeds can absorb up to 12 times their weight. This ability is primarily due to the soluble fiber present in the seeds. Soluble fiber forms a gel-like substance in the digestive tract, which slows the digestion process. This can help stabilize blood sugar levels, increase satiety, and improve overall nutrient absorption.

The gelatinous consistency of soluble fiber also plays a crucial role in promoting bowel regularity. It helps soften stools, making them easier to pass, thus relieving constipation. For those suffering from irregular bowel movements, incorporating chia seeds into the diet can provide much-needed relief.

Insoluble Fiber: The Gut's Best Friend

Insoluble fiber, on the other hand, adds bulk to the stool and promotes regular bowel movements by speeding up transit time through the digestive system. Chia seeds contain significant amounts of insoluble fiber, contributing to their reputation as a gut-friendly digestive aid.

A diet rich in insoluble fiber can help prevent constipation and reduce the risk of developing digestive disorders such as hemorrhoids and diverticulitis. By including chia seeds in your meals, you not only support regularity but also promote a healthier intestinal environment.

Prebiotic Properties

In addition to their fiber content, chia seeds have prebiotic properties that can significantly enhance digestive health. Prebiotics are compounds in food that induce the growth or activity of beneficial microorganisms, particularly in the gut. They act as food for probiotics, the good bacteria that play an essential role in maintaining gut health.

Chia seeds help nourish these beneficial bacteria, promoting a balanced microbiome. A healthy gut microbiome is associated with better digestion, improved immune function, and even better mental health. By nurturing gut flora, chia seeds contribute to a holistic approach to digestive well-being.

Weight Management and Digestion

Another way chia seeds contribute to digestive health is through their role in weight management. Their high fiber content increases feelings of fullness, which can help reduce overall caloric intake. When you feel satisfied after a meal, you're less likely to indulge in unhealthy snacks, thus promoting better digestive health by minimizing overeating.

Moreover, the slow digestion encouraged by the gel-like structure of soluble fiber can help maintain stable energy levels, preventing the blood sugar spikes and crashes that often lead to cravings and subsequent digestive distress.

Practical Applications

Incorporating chia seeds into your diet is a seamless and versatile way to enhance your digestive health. Here are some practical applications:

Chia Pudding: Combine chia seeds with your favorite milk or plant-based alternative, add sweeteners, and let the mixture sit overnight. The next day, you'll have a delicious, creamy pudding that's rich in fiber.

Smoothies: Add a tablespoon of chia seeds to your daily smoothie. They blend well with fruits, vegetables, and other ingredients, providing an added nutrient boost.

Baking: Incorporate chia seeds into muffins, breads, and other baked goods. They can act as a binding agent while enhancing the fiber content.

Salads: Sprinkle chia seeds on top of salads or mix them into dressings for added texture and nutrition.

Gel Substitute for Egg: In vegan baking, chia seeds can be used as an egg substitute. Mixing one tablespoon of chia seeds with three tablespoons of water creates a gel that functions as a binder in recipes.

Chia seeds are more than just a trendy ingredient; they are an ancient food with powerful digestive benefits. Their high fiber content, prebiotic properties, and role in promoting feelings of satisfaction make them an excellent addition to any diet aimed at enhancing digestive health. As we move forward in our exploration of superfoods, it is clear that embracing chia seeds may not only support digestion but also foster a balanced lifestyle.

Fiber Content and Its Role chia seeds

This chapter explores the significance of fiber in chia seeds, elucidating its different types, health impacts, and the unique attributes that make chia seeds an invaluable addition to our diets.

The Composition of Chia Seeds

Chia seeds (Salvia hispanica) are tiny black or white seeds derived from the flowering plant native to Central and South America. Often touted as a superfood, these tiny seeds are packed with nutrients, one of the most notable being fiber. A single ounce (about 28 grams) of chia seeds contains approximately 10 grams of dietary fiber, representing a striking 40% of their total weight. This fiber is primarily soluble, meaning it absorbs water and forms a gel-like substance, which plays a significant role in digestive health and overall well-being.

Types of Fiber in Chia Seeds

Soluble Fiber: This type of fiber dissolves in water, forming a viscous gel. Soluble fiber is highly beneficial for regulating blood sugar levels and reducing cholesterol. In chia seeds, soluble fiber contributes to the feeling of fullness, helping to control appetite and manage weight effectively.

Insoluble Fiber: Unlike soluble fiber, insoluble fiber does not dissolve in water. Instead, it adds bulk to stool and aids in the movement of food through the digestive tract. Although chia seeds contain less insoluble fiber compared to soluble fiber, the presence of both types ensures a balanced approach to digestive health.

Health Benefits of Dietary Fiber in Chia Seeds

The inclusion of chia seeds in the diet offers a myriad of health benefits attributed to their high fiber content. Here, we delve into some of the key advantages.

1. Digestive Health

One of the foremost benefits of dietary fiber is its impact on digestive health. Chia seeds, with their rich fiber composition, promote regular bowel movements and alleviate issues such as constipation. The soluble fiber component aids in forming a gel-like substance that helps smooth digestion, while the insoluble fiber enhances overall gut health.

2. Blood Sugar Regulation

Soluble fiber is instrumental in moderating the absorption of sugar in the bloodstream, which can prevent spikes in blood sugar levels. This characteristic of chia seeds makes them an excellent food choice for individuals managing diabetes or those seeking to maintain stable energy levels throughout the day.

3. Weight Management

Chia seeds are often regarded as a weight-loss-friendly food due to their ability to absorb up to twelve times their weight in water. When soaked, they expand and create a sense of fullness that may help reduce overall calorie intake. Additionally, the presence of fiber aids in prolonged satiety, curbing unnecessary snacking and promoting healthier eating habits.

4. Heart Health

The fiber found in chia seeds can positively influence heart health. By lowering cholesterol levels and improving blood pressure, a higher intake of dietary fiber is associated with a reduced risk of cardiovascular diseases. Additionally, the omega-3 fatty acids present in chia seeds complement their fiber content to support overall heart health.

Incorporating Chia Seeds into the Diet

Given their unique properties and health benefits, incorporating chia seeds into one's diet can be a simple yet effective way to boost fiber intake. Here are a few suggestions:

Smoothies: Blend chia seeds into your morning smoothie for added nutrition and thickness.

Oatmeal: Stir in chia seeds into oatmeal or porridge for a fiber boost.

Baked Goods: Add grounded chia seeds to muffins, bread, or pancakes.

Salads: Sprinkle whole chia seeds on top of salads for a crunchy texture.

Soaking chia seeds in water or plant-based milk can also

enhance their digestibility and make a great base for puddings or dressings.

As more people become aware of the importance of dietary fiber and its role in overall health, chia seeds are likely to remain a staple in health-conscious diets around the world. Embracing these tiny seeds can pave the way for a nutritious and balanced lifestyle, emphasizing the timeless saying that great things often come in small packages.

Hydration and Gel Formation in chia seeds

One remarkable characteristic that distinguishes chia seeds from other seeds is their ability to absorb water and form a gel-like substance when hydrated. This chapter delves into the science behind hydration and gel formation in chia seeds, exploring the mechanisms, benefits, and culinary applications of this unique phenomenon.

The Science of Hydration

Chia seeds have a high fiber content, consisting primarily of soluble fiber, which plays a crucial role in their hydration capability. When chia seeds come into contact with water, they can absorb up to 12 times their weight due to their hydrophilic properties. This process begins with the absorption of water through the hard outer shell of the seeds.

The Role of Soluble Fiber

Soluble fiber, primarily composed of mucilage, is the key component responsible for the gel formation in chia seeds.

Mucilage is a viscous substance that swells and creates a gel when it interacts with water. As the chia seeds are immersed in water, the soluble fiber draws in moisture and swells, creating a thick, gel-like coating around each seed.

The Hydration Process

The hydration process can be divided into several stages:

Initial Contact: When chia seeds are introduced to water, the outer membrane begins to absorb moisture almost immediately.

Swelling: As the seeds continue to absorb water, they increase in size and the mucilage begins to expand, forming a viscous gel.

Equilibrium: After a period of time, usually about 30 minutes to two hours, the seeds reach a state of equilibrium, where they have absorbed maximum water and are surrounded by a gel matrix. The exact time required may vary based on the temperature of the water and the seed itself.

Stability: The gel retains its structure quite well, making it a stable medium for various culinary applications.

Gel Formation Mechanism

The mechanical properties of the gel formed from chia seeds are attributed to the interplay between water and the hydrophilic constituents of the soluble fiber. The structure of the mucilage allows it to form a network that traps water molecules, resulting in a stable gel. This phenomenon is also related to the seed's lipid profile, which includes omega-3 fatty acids, further enhancing its health benefits.

Factors Influencing Gel Formation

Several factors influence the extent and nature of gel formation in chia seeds:

Water Temperature: Warm water can expedite the swelling process, while cold water may slow it down.

Hydration Time: A longer soaking period increases gel formation, allowing for more thorough hydration.

Seed Size: The size of chia seeds can influence the rate of hydration; smaller seeds tend to absorb water more quickly.

Concentration: The ratio of chia seeds to water affects the viscosity of the gel formed; a higher seed concentration results in a thicker gel.

Nutritional and Health Benefits

The gel-forming ability of chia seeds adds several nutritional benefits:

Satiety: The gel expands in the stomach, promoting a feeling of fullness and aiding in weight management.

Blood Sugar Regulation: The soluble fiber can slow down the absorption of carbohydrates, leading to better blood sugar control.

Digestive Health: The fiber content helps maintain healthy digestion and regular bowel movements.

Hydration: The gel retains water, making chia seeds a valuable addition to hydration strategies, especially in hot climates or during physical activity.

Culinary Applications

Chia seeds are versatile ingredients in the culinary world, primarily due to their unique gel formation. Here are some popular applications:

Chia Pudding: One of the most well-known uses, chia seeds are soaked in milk or a milk alternative, combined with sweeteners and flavorings, resulting in a creamy pudding.

Thickening Agent: The gel can act as a natural thickener in smoothies, soups, or sauces, imparting a smooth texture without the need for added starches.

Egg Substitute: In vegan cooking, the gel formed from chia seeds can substitute for eggs in recipes, providing binding properties in baked goods.

Toppings and Mix-ins: The gel can be added to yogurt, oatmeal, or salads, providing a nutritious boost and an interesting texture.

Understanding the science behind this process not only highlights the health advantages associated with chia seeds but also inspires innovative culinary applications. As interest in plant-based nutrition continues to rise, chia seeds stand out as a superfood, offering a unique blend of functionality and health benefits. Future research may further unravel the intricacies of chia seed hydration, potentially unlocking new avenues for their use in health and nutrition.

Chapter 4: Introducing Chia Seeds to Your Child's Diet

Rich in omega-3 fatty acids, fiber, protein, and various micronutrients, chia seeds offer a multitude of health benefits that can support your child's growth and development. This chapter will guide you through the nutritional benefits of chia seeds, how to introduce them into your child's meals, and creative ways to make them appealing.

Understanding the Nutritional Benefits of Chia Seeds

Before diving into how to incorporate chia seeds into your child's diet, it's essential to understand what makes them so nutritious. Here are some of the key benefits:

1. Rich in Omega-3 Fatty Acids

Chia seeds are one of the richest plant-based sources of omega-3 fatty acids, which are crucial for brain health and development. Increasing omega-3 intake can promote cognitive function, which is particularly important during early childhood and adolescence.

2. High in Fiber

Chia seeds are incredibly high in fiber, which can help maintain digestive health. A fiber-rich diet can prevent constipation, promote a feeling of fullness, and even contribute to a healthy weight. With appropriately small servings, chia seeds can be an excellent way to help children feel full after meals.

3. Protein Powerhouse

Chia seeds contain more than 20% protein by weight,

making them an excellent source of plant-based protein. Protein is vital for growth, muscle development, and overall health, especially for active children.

4. Packed with Nutrients

These tiny seeds are loaded with essential vitamins and minerals such as calcium, magnesium, phosphorus, and iron. These nutrients support bone health and the immune system, making chia seeds a fantastic addition to a child's diet.

How to Introduce Chia Seeds to Your Child

Introducing chia seeds into your child's diet doesn't have to be complicated or intimidating. Here are some simple strategies to seamlessly integrate chia into their meals.

1. Start Slowly

If your child is new to chia seeds, start with small amounts. Adding a teaspoon to meals can be a good starting point. As they become accustomed to the taste and texture, gradually increase the amount.

2. **Mix into Smoothies**

Smoothies are a fantastic way to introduce chia seeds because they blend in well with other flavors. Simply add a teaspoon of chia seeds to your child's favorite smoothie recipe. The seeds will add nutrition without affecting the taste.

3. **Incorporate into Oatmeal or Yogurt**

Sprinkling chia seeds onto oatmeal or mixing them into yogurt can create a nutritious breakfast or snack. Combine them with fruits, honey, or nut butter to make it more enticing.

4. **Baking with Chia Seeds**

When baking muffins, pancakes, or quick breads, you can easily incorporate chia seeds. They can be added directly to the batter or used as an egg substitute by mixing one tablespoon of chia seeds with three tablespoons of water and letting it sit until it forms a gel-like consistency.

5. **Create Chia Pudding**

Chia pudding is an excellent way to showcase the versatility of chia seeds. Simply combine chia seeds, milk (or a non-dairy alternative), and a sweetener, then let it sit in the refrigerator for a few hours or overnight.

You can customize it by adding vanilla extract, cocoa powder, or layering it with fruit. The texture can be fun for kids, and it feels like a dessert!

6. **Use in Soups and Sauces**

If your child enjoys soups and sauces, consider adding chia seeds to them. They can be blended into the mixture or stirred in while cooking. This is a stealthy way to enhance the nutritional value of everyday meals.

Making Chia Seeds Appealing

One of the challenges parents face is making healthful foods appealing to children. Here are a few creative ideas to make chia seeds a fun part of your child's diet:

1. **Colorful Presentation**

Children eat with their eyes first. Use colorful fruits and toppings to make meals vibrant. For instance, serve chia pudding in a clear glass layered with fresh strawberries and blueberries for visual appeal.

2. **Involve Your Child**

Let your children help with meal preparation. They can sprinkle chia seeds into smoothies, help measure them for baking, or mix them into yogurt. Making them part of the process can increase their interest in trying new foods.

3. **Tell a Story**

Children are often more willing to try new foods when there's a story behind them. Share the adventure of how chia seeds were used by ancient cultures and how they can be part of their growth and health.

4. **Fun Names**

Creating a fun name for dishes containing chia seeds can make meal times more exciting. For example, calling chia pudding "magic jelly" might capture your child's imagination.

5. **Experiment with Textures**

Chia seeds can be either crunchy or gel-like, depending on how they're prepared. Some children prefer the crunch, while others may like the pudding-like consistency. Experiment to find what your child enjoys most.

Safe Dosages and Recommendations When Using Chia Seeds for Children

However, when it comes to incorporating chia seeds into the diets of children, it is essential for parents and caregivers to understand the appropriate dosages, potential benefits, and any potential concerns.

Understanding Chia Seeds

Chia seeds, derived from the Salvia hispanica plant, are

native to Mexico and Guatemala. Historically, they were a staple food for ancient civilizations such as the Aztecs and Mayans, revered for their ability to provide sustained energy. In recent years, they have become included in modern diets, often marketed as a superfood.

The seeds have a unique ability to absorb water—up to 12 times their weight—forming a gel-like consistency when soaked. This characteristic not only enhances their nutritional value but also aids digestion and promotes a feeling of fullness.

Nutritional Benefits for Children ### 1. Heart Health

Chia seeds are an excellent source of alpha-linolenic acid (ALA), a type of omega-3 fatty acid that supports

heart health and overall well-being. Including this nutrient in a child's diet can contribute to improved cardiovascular function.

2. Digestive Health

Given their high fiber content, chia seeds can promote healthy digestion. Fiber is essential for regulating bowel movements and preventing constipation, a common issue in children.

3. Protein Source

Chia seeds contain a decent amount of plant-based protein, making them an excellent addition to vegetarian or vegan diets. Protein is crucial for growth and tissue repair, especially during childhood.

4. Calcium and Other Minerals

Chia seeds are a good source of calcium, magnesium, and phosphorus, which are important for bone health and development in growing children.

Recommended Dosages

When introducing chia seeds into a child's diet, it is crucial to adhere to recommended dosage guidelines to ensure safety and avoid any adverse effects.

1. Age Appropriateness

Ages 1-3: Start with small amounts, about 1 teaspoon (5 grams) of soaked chia seeds per day. It's important to ensure children can adequately chew and digest the seeds, or they can be blended into smoothies or yogurt.

Ages 4-8: Increase the dosage to about 1-2 tablespoons (15-30 grams) of soaked chia seeds per day. As children's digestive systems mature, they can handle larger quantities.

Ages 9-12: The dosage can be further increased to 2-3 tablespoons (30-45 grams) daily. It's essential to ensure that they remain hydrated, as chia seeds can absorb a significant amount of water.

2. Gradual Introduction

When introducing chia seeds into a child's diet, it's crucial to start with small amounts to assess tolerance. Gradually increase the dosage while monitoring for any digestive issues, such as bloating or discomfort.

3. Proper Preparation

Chia seeds should be soaked in liquid—water, milk, or yogurt—for at least 30 minutes before consumption. This process allows the seeds to expand and helps minimize the risk of choking. Soaked chia seeds can be added to various dishes, including smoothies, oatmeal, pancakes, and salads.

Potential Concerns

While chia seeds are considered safe for most children, there are some potential concerns to be aware of: ### 1. Allergies

Though rare, some individuals may be allergic to chia seeds. Parents should monitor for any signs of an allergic reaction, such as rash, swelling, or difficulty breathing, particularly when introducing the seeds for the first time.

2. Digestive Issues

If consumed in large quantities without adequate hydration, chia seeds can lead to digestive issues, including constipation or bloating. Ensure children drink plenty of fluids when incorporating chia seeds into their meals.

3. Supervision During Consumption

For younger children, parental supervision during meals is advised to prevent choking hazards. Ensure that chia seeds are appropriately prepared and served in a manageable form.

Always consult a pediatrician or a registered dietitian if there are any questions or concerns regarding a child's diet and the introduction of new foods. Encouraging children to explore a diverse array of foods, including superfoods like chia seeds, can pave the way for a lifetime of healthy eating habits.

Creative Ways to Include Chia Seeds for Kids

As parents, finding nutritious ingredients that children enjoy can sometimes feel like a daunting task. However, chia seeds offer a versatile solution to enhance your child's diet in engaging and enjoyable ways. This chapter will explore creative ideas to incorporate chia seeds into meals and snacks, ensuring your kids receive the health benefits without fuss.

Understanding Chia Seeds

Before diving into the creative ideas, let's take a moment to understand why chia seeds are excellent for children. These tiny seeds are rich in:

Omega-3 Fatty Acids: Beneficial for brain health and development.

Fiber: Promotes digestive health and helps keep kids full.

Protein: Essential for growth and muscle development.

Calcium, Iron, and Antioxidants: Important for overall health.

Their neutral flavor and gelatinous texture when soaked allow chia seeds to blend seamlessly into various dishes.

1. Chia Pudding: A Fun Breakfast or Snack

Chia pudding is a fantastic way to include chia seeds in your kid's diet. It's simple to make and can be flavored in multiple ways to cater to your child's taste preferences.

Basic Chia Pudding Recipe:

Ingredients:

1/4 cup chia seeds

1 cup almond milk (or any milk of choice)

1 tablespoon honey or maple syrup (optional)

1/2 teaspoon vanilla extract

Fresh fruits, nuts, or granola for toppings

Instructions:

In a bowl, combine chia seeds, milk, sweetener, and vanilla extract.

Stir well to prevent clumping.

Let it sit for about 15 minutes, then stir again. Refrigerate for 2 hours or overnight until it thickens.

Serve with your child's favorite toppings.

Variations: Add cocoa powder for chocolate lovers, or fruit purees for a fruity twist. Allow your kids to choose their toppings for a fun DIY breakfast.

2. Chia-Infused Smoothies

Smoothies are an excellent vehicle for sneaking in nutrition. Chia seeds can boost a smoothie's nutritional profile without altering its taste.

Berry Chia Smoothie:

Ingredients:

1 cup frozen mixed berries

1 banana

1 cup spinach (optional)

1 cup yogurt or plant-based yogurt

1 tablespoon chia seeds

1 cup juice or milk

Instructions:

Blend all ingredients until smooth.

Serve immediately. Allow kids to add a straw for fun flair.

Tip: Let kids pick their favorites from a selection of fruits and greens. This choice engages them and teaches them about nutrition.

3. Chia Seed Pancakes or Waffles

Transform breakfast into an exciting affair by incorporating chia seeds into pancakes or waffles. They'll never guess how healthy these treats are!

Chia Pancakes Recipe:

Ingredients:

1 cup flour (whole wheat or regular)

1 tablespoon baking powder

1 tablespoon chia seeds

1 tablespoon sugar (optional)

1 cup milk

1 egg

2 tablespoons melted butter or oil

Pinch of salt

Instructions:

Combine all dry ingredients in one bowl and wet ingredients in another.

Mix together until smooth.

Pour onto a heated skillet and cook until bubbles form, then flip.

Serving Suggestion: Serve with fresh fruit, yogurt, or a drizzle of maple syrup. The chia seeds add a subtle crunch that's delightful!

4. Chia Seed Jellies or Jams

Making homemade jellies or jams is an exciting activity for kids. Chia seeds can replace pectin, giving a nutritious twist to your spread.

Simple Chia Jam:

Ingredients:

2 cups of your favorite fruits (like strawberries or blueberries)

2 tablespoons honey or maple syrup (optional)

2 tablespoons chia seeds

Instructions:

Blend the fruits until smooth.

Mix in honey and chia seeds.

Let it sit for about 15-30 minutes to thicken.

Pair It With: Spread this jam on toast, yogurt, or pancakes for a sweet treat packed with nutrients! #### 5. Fun Snacks with Chia Seeds

Incorporating chia seeds doesn't have to be limited to meals. They can easily be added to snacks, making healthy munching fun for kids.

Chia Seed Energy Bites:

Ingredients:

1 cup rolled oats

1/2 cup nut butter

1/4 cup honey or maple syrup

1/4 cup chia seeds

1/4 cup chocolate chips (optional)

Instructions:

Mix all ingredients in a bowl until combined.

Roll into small balls and place them on a baking sheet.

Refrigerate for about 30 minutes before serving.

These energy bites can be a perfect after-school snack that will keep kids energized and satisfied.

The ideas shared in this chapter are just the beginning—feel free to experiment and get creative with these tiny powerhouses. By involving your children in the process—whether it's picking toppings for chia pudding or mixing ingredients for jam—you'll create not just healthy meals but also delightful moments in the kitchen. Embrace the versatility of chia seeds, and watch your kids thrive as they enjoy yummy, wholesome treats!

Chapter 5: Tasty Chia Seed Recipes for Kids

Luckily, chia seeds can be incorporated into a variety of delicious and nutritious recipes that even the pickiest eaters will enjoy. In this chapter, we'll explore some fun and tasty chia seed recipes perfect for kids!

1. Chia Pudding Parfait ### Ingredients:

1/4 cup chia seeds

1 cup almond milk (or any milk of choice)

1 tablespoon honey or maple syrup (optional)

1/2 teaspoon vanilla extract

Fresh fruit (e.g., strawberries, blueberries, bananas)

Granola

Instructions:

In a mixing bowl, combine chia seeds, almond milk, honey (if using), and vanilla extract. Stir well to ensure the chia seeds are evenly distributed.

Let the mixture sit for about 10 minutes, then stir again to break up any clumps. Refrigerate for at least 2 hours or overnight for the best results.

When ready to serve, layer the chia pudding in a cup or bowl with fresh fruit and a sprinkle of granola on top. Create fun layers and let your kids pick their favorite fruit combinations!

Fun Tip:

Let your kids help assemble the parfaits! They can choose

which fruits to add and how to layer them, making it a fun and engaging activity.

2. Chia Seed Smoothie ### Ingredients:

1 tablespoon chia seeds

1 banana

1/2 cup spinach (optional but nutritious!)

1/2 cup yogurt (plain or flavored)

1 cup milk (or milk alternative)

1 tablespoon peanut butter or almond butter

Honey to taste (optional)

Instructions:

In a blender, combine all ingredients and blend until smooth.

If the consistency is too thick, add a splash more milk to reach your desired texture.

Pour it into a fun cup and enjoy with a straw!

Fun Tip:

Have a smoothie-making party! Lay out various ingredients and let kids customize their smoothies. Offer toppings like chia seeds, shredded coconut, or chocolate chips for extra flair.

3. Chia Seed Energy Bites ### Ingredients:

1 cup rolled oats

1/2 cup nut butter (peanut, almond, or sunflower seed)

1/4 cup honey or maple syrup

1/4 cup chia seeds

1/4 cup mini chocolate chips

1/4 cup raisins or dried fruit

1 teaspoon vanilla extract

Instructions:

In a mixing bowl, combine all ingredients and stir until well-mixed.

Use your hands to form the mixture into small balls, about the size of a tablespoon.

Place the energy bites on a baking sheet lined with parchment paper and refrigerate for 30 minutes until firm. Store them in an airtight container in the fridge.

Fun Tip:

Get creative with the mix-ins! Your children can add their favorite ingredients like shredded coconut, sunflower seeds, or even a pinch of cinnamon.

4. Chia Seed Pancakes ### Ingredients:

1 cup whole wheat flour

2 tablespoons chia seeds

2 tablespoons sugar or sweetener of choice

1 tablespoon baking powder

1/2 teaspoon salt

1 cup milk

1 egg

2 tablespoons melted butter or coconut oil

Optional: Fresh berries for topping

Instructions:

In a bowl, mix together the flour, chia seeds, sugar, baking powder, and salt.

In a separate bowl, whisk together the milk, egg, and melted butter.

Combine the wet and dry ingredients, stirring until just blended; the batter will be thick.

Heat a non-stick skillet over medium heat and pour in 1/4 cup of batter for each pancake. Cook until bubbles form on the surface, then flip and cook until golden brown.

Serve warm with fresh berries and a drizzle of maple syrup.

Fun Tip:

Let kids get involved in the cooking process! They can help with whisking, pouring, and flipping pancakes (with supervision) to make breakfast a family affair.

5. Chia Seed Jam ### Ingredients:

2 cups berries (fresh or frozen)

2 tablespoons chia seeds

2-3 tablespoons honey or maple syrup

1 tablespoon lemon juice

Instructions:

In a saucepan over medium heat, combine the berries and lemon juice. Cook down for about 5-10 minutes until the berries are soft and start breaking apart.

Remove from heat and stir in the chia seeds and sweetener. Mix well until combined.

Allow the mixture to cool before placing it in a jar. Refrigerate for up to one week.

Fun Tip:

Use the chia seed jam to smear on toast, mix into yogurt, or as a topping for pancakes. Kids can explore different flavors by mixing various berries!

Involving your children in the preparation and letting them choose their favorite flavors can make them more excited about trying new foods. Whether it's a colorful parfait, a refreshing smoothie, or tasty pancakes, these recipes are sure to become family favorites! Enjoy the nutritious journey together!

Breakfast Boosters including Chia Seeds for Kids

To make breakfast as nutritious as possible, incorporating foods packed with vitamins, minerals, fiber, and healthy fats can create a powerful morning meal. One superfood that has gained popularity in recent years is chia seeds. This chapter explores how breakfast boosters, including chia seeds, can enhance the morning routine of children.

The Importance of Breakfast

Before diving into the specifics, let's take a moment to understand why breakfast is crucial for children. After a night of fasting, kids wake up with their bodies in need of fuel. Breakfast helps replenish energy stores and can improve cognitive function, mood, and physical performance. Research has consistently shown that children who eat a nutritious breakfast fare better in school, demonstrate improved concentration, and show better behavior throughout their day.

Introducing Chia Seeds

Chia seeds are tiny, nutrient-dense seeds that come from the Salvia hispanica plant, native to Mexico. They are an excellent source of omega-3 fatty acids, fiber, antioxidants, and essential minerals such as calcium, magnesium, and iron. The tiny seeds are unique; when soaked in liquid, they expand and turn gelatinous, which can add interesting texture to meals.

Given their nutrient profile, chia seeds make an excellent addition to breakfast, particularly for children whose bodies are still growing and developing. They can help keep kids fuller for longer, thanks to their high fiber content, and can aid in regulating blood sugar levels, preventing the energy crashes often experienced after sugary breakfast options.

Creative Ways to Incorporate Chia Seeds into Breakfast

Here are several fun and easy ways to include chia seeds into your child's breakfast, making sure it's both delicious and nutritious:

1. **Chia Pudding**

Chia pudding is a versatile and delicious breakfast option that can be prepared the night before. Simply combine chia seeds with milk (dairy or plant-based), a touch of sweetener like honey or maple syrup, and flavorings such as vanilla or cocoa. Let the mixture sit in the fridge overnight, and by morning, you'll have a creamy pudding. Kids can customize their pudding with toppings like fruits, nuts, or granola.

Recipe Idea: Berry Chia Pudding

1/4 cup chia seeds

1 cup almond milk (or milk of choice)

1 tablespoon honey or maple syrup

1/2 teaspoon vanilla extract

Fresh berries for topping

Mix all ingredients in a jar, shake well, and refrigerate overnight. Serve topped with fresh berries in the morning.

2. **Chia Seed Smoothies**

Smoothies are another excellent way to sneak in chia seeds. Blend their favorite fruits with yogurt or milk and add a tablespoon of chia seeds for an extra nutrient boost. This is an ideal breakfast for kids on the go.

Recipe Idea: Tropical Chia Smoothie

1 banana

1/2 cup pineapple chunks

1 cup spinach (optional)

1 tablespoon chia seeds

1 cup coconut water or milk

Blend until smooth and serve immediately. #### 3. **Chia-Infused Oatmeal**

Oatmeal is a breakfast classic, and adding chia seeds takes it to the next level. Stir in chia seeds while cooking the oats, or sprinkle them on top before serving. This adds a delightful crunch and an added nutritional boost.

Recipe Idea: Banana Chia Oatmeal

1 cup rolled oats

2 cups water or milk

1 ripe banana, mashed

2 tablespoons chia seeds

Cinnamon to taste

Optional: nuts or chocolate chips

Cook the oats according to package instructions. Stir in mashed banana and spices, then top with chia seeds and any other favorites.

4. **Chia Seed Pancakes**

Transform an ordinary pancake breakfast into an extraordinary one by adding chia seeds to the batter. Not only does it enhance the nutritional value, but it also gives pancakes an appealing texture and subtle crunch.

Recipe Idea: Chia Pancakes

1 cup whole wheat flour

1 tablespoon baking powder

1 tablespoon chia seeds

1 cup milk

1 egg

1 tablespoon maple syrup

Mix dry ingredients in one bowl and wet ingredients in

another, then combine. Cook on a skillet and serve with fresh fruit and syrup.

Tips for Kids to Enjoy Chia Seeds

Get Them Involved: Involve kids in breakfast preparation to create excitement around trying new foods. Let them choose toppings for chia pudding or select fruits for smoothies.

Make It Fun: Create fun names for dishes, like "Superhero Chia Pudding" or "Rocket Fuel Smoothie," to encourage kids to taste them.

Start Small: If introducing chia seeds for the first time, start with smaller amounts to see how kids enjoy the texture and taste.

Experiment: Try different combinations of flavors and textures to keep breakfast a delightful experience that kids look forward to.

Incorporating chia seeds into breakfast is just one way to boost the nutritional value of your child's morning meal. By providing them with energy-dense, nutrient-rich foods, you can help cultivate healthy eating habits that will carry into their adult lives. Don't be afraid to experiment with variations and recipes, keeping breakfast both nutritious and enjoyable. With breakfast boosters like chia seeds, you're setting your child on a path to success, one delicious bite at a time.

Snack Time Favorites Including Chia Seeds for Kids

It's a moment to recharge, explore new flavors, and enjoy food in a fun and relaxed setting. In this chapter, we'll explore exciting and nutritious snack ideas that incorporate chia seeds—tiny powerhouses of nutrition—making even the simplest snack time a celebratory event!

The Nutritional Power of Chia Seeds

Chia seeds may be small in size, but they are mighty in nutrition. Packed with omega-3 fatty acids, fiber, protein, and various essential minerals, chia seeds are an excellent addition to your child's diet. These tiny seeds can help promote digestive health, provide sustained energy, and support overall wellness. Best of all, they're incredibly versatile and can be added to various recipes without altering the taste too much.

Fun and Easy Chia Seed Snack Ideas

Now let's dive into some delicious and child-approved snack ideas that incorporate chia seeds. From smoothies to treats, these options are sure to please even the pickiest of eaters.

1. Chia Seed Pudding

Ingredients:

1/4 cup chia seeds

1 cup milk (dairy or non-dairy)

1-2 tablespoons sweetener (honey, maple syrup, or agave)

1/2 teaspoon vanilla extract

Toppings: fresh fruit, nuts, or granola

Instructions:

In a bowl, combine chia seeds, milk, sweetener, and vanilla extract.

Mix well, ensuring that the chia seeds are evenly distributed.

Let the mixture sit for 5-10 minutes, then stir again to prevent clumping.

Cover and refrigerate for at least 2 hours or overnight until it thickens to a pudding-like consistency.

Before serving, let your kids choose their favorite toppings. They can customize their pudding with fruits like berries, bananas, or mango, adding a delightful touch of color and flavor.

2. Chia Seed Fruit Snacks

Ingredients:

1 cup fruit juice (100% natural, no added sugar)

2 tablespoons chia seeds

Optional: pureed fruit for added flavor

Instructions:

In a small bowl, combine the fruit juice and chia seeds.

Stir well and let it sit for 10-15 minutes, allowing the chia seeds to absorb the liquid and swell.

Once the mixture thickens, pour it into silicone molds or an ice cube tray.

Freeze for a few hours until solid.

Pop out the snacks and store them in a bag in the freezer for a refreshing treat!

3. Chia Seed Granola Bars

Ingredients:

2 cups rolled oats

1/2 cup honey or maple syrup

1/2 cup nut butter (peanut, almond, or sunflower seed butter)

1/4 cup chia seeds

1/2 cup mix-ins (dried fruit, chocolate chips, nuts)

Instructions:

Preheat the oven to 350°F (175°C) and line an 8x8 inch baking dish with parchment paper.

In a large mixing bowl, combine oats, chia seeds, nut butter, and honey. Mix well until everything is combined.

Fold in the mix-ins of your choice.

Press the mixture firmly into the prepared baking dish.

Bake for 15-20 minutes, or until the edges are golden brown.

Allow to cool before cutting into squares. These granola bars make for a perfect on-the-go snack! #### 4. Chia Seed Smoothie

Ingredients:

1 cup milk or yogurt

1 ripe banana

1/2 cup spinach (optional for added nutrients)

2 tablespoons chia seeds

1 tablespoon honey or agave (optional)

Instructions:

In a blender, combine all the ingredients until smooth.

If you want a thicker consistency, add more chia seeds and let the smoothie sit for a few minutes to allow the seeds to bloom.

Serve in a fun cup or jar, and maybe add a colorful straw for extra flair! ### Making Snack Time Fun

We all know that kids eat with their eyes first. To make snack time even more appealing, get creative with colors, shapes, and presentations. Use cookie cutters to create fun shapes from fruits and homemade treats, or have a "build your own" snack bar where children can assemble their snacks using various ingredients. Engaging kids in the kitchen also helps them develop a positive relationship with food and encourages healthy eating habits.

By incorporating chia seeds into fun snack ideas, you can provide your children with delicious treats that are not only tasty but also nutrient-dense. So, gather the ingredients, invite your kids to help in the kitchen, and enjoy these scrumptious snacks together—they're sure to become favorites for snack time!

Chapter 6: Hydration and Its Importance for Constipation

While several factors contribute to constipation, including diet, lifestyle, and stress, one crucial aspect often overlooked is hydration. In this chapter, we will explore the importance of hydration in maintaining gut health, the role chia seeds can play in alleviating constipation, and how these two elements synergistically improve digestive function.

The Role of Hydration in Digestive Health

Water is an essential component of various biological processes and plays a particularly vital role in digestion. The human body is composed of approximately 60% water, highlighting its importance in maintaining life and overall health. For optimal digestive function, proper hydration is crucial for several reasons:

Softens Stools

Water helps soften stools, making them easier to pass through the intestines. When the body is dehydrated, the colon absorbs more water from waste material, resulting in harder, drier stools that are difficult to eliminate.

Facilitates Digestion

Hydration aids the proper function of enzymes necessary for breaking down food in the digestive tract. Without sufficient water, digestive enzymes can become less effective, slowing the digestive process.

Promotes Regularity

Adequate fluid intake helps ensure the smooth movement

of food through the gastrointestinal tract. By keeping things moving, hydration plays a key role in maintaining regular bowel movements.

Prevents Constipation

When the body is well-hydrated, the chances of developing constipation decrease significantly. Hydrated muscles are better able to contract and relax, helping to push stools through the intestines effectively.

Chia Seeds: A Nutritional Powerhouse

Chia seeds have gained popularity in recent years as a superfood due to their rich nutritional profile. These tiny seeds, derived from the Salvia hispanica plant, are packed with essential nutrients, including:

Fiber

Chia seeds are an excellent source of dietary fiber, particularly soluble fiber. Soluble fiber absorbs water and forms a gel-like substance in the gut, aiding digestion and promoting regularity.

Omega-3 Fatty Acids

Chia seeds are rich in alpha-linolenic acid (ALA), a type of omega-3 fatty acid that is beneficial for overall health and can reduce intestinal inflammation.

Antioxidants

These seeds contain antioxidants that help combat oxidative stress and may support gut health by preventing damage to the digestive lining.

Hydrophilic Properties

Chia seeds can absorb up to 12 times their weight in water,

swelling to form a gel-like consistency when hydrated. This unique characteristic not only enhances their health benefits but also aids in hydration.

The Synergy of Hydration and Chia Seeds

The combination of proper hydration and the incorporation of chia seeds into one's diet can significantly improve digestive health and alleviate constipation. Here's how they work together:

Enhanced Stool Softening: When chia seeds are consumed, the soluble fiber they contain swells and absorbs water. This process creates bulk in the stool while also effectively softening it, making it easier to pass. For those struggling with constipation, incorporating chia seeds into a balanced diet can lead to significant improvements.

Increased Fluid Intake: Chia seeds can serve as a reminder to increase fluid intake. Since these seeds absorb water, they encourage individuals to drink more fluids throughout the day to ensure optimal texture and consistency of the gel formed in the gut. This relationship between chia seeds and hydration can lead to a more conscious effort to meet daily fluid recommendations.

Balanced Nutrition: Chia seeds are versatile and can be easily added to various meals and snacks. Whether mixed into smoothies, sprinkled on salads, or used in baking, they provide both fiber and hydration benefits, making them an accessible addition to a high-fiber diet aimed at alleviating constipation.

Regular Consumption: One of the keys to effective management of constipation is the regular incorporation of high-fiber foods in the diet. When paired with adequate hydration, chia seeds can be a part of a consistent routine that promotes gut health and digestive efficiency.

How to Incorporate Chia Seeds for Optimal Hydration

To harness the benefits of chia seeds alongside proper hydration, consider the following tips:

Soak Before Use: Before consuming chia seeds, soak them in water or your favorite beverage for about 30 minutes. This allows the seeds to expand and create a gel-like consistency, enhancing their hydrating properties.

Add to Beverages: Mix soaked chia seeds into juices, teas, or smoothies for added texture and nutrition. This easily integrates hydration with the benefits of fiber.

Mix into Foods: Incorporate chia seeds into yogurt, oatmeal, or baked goods. This way, you can enjoy the health benefits while staying hydrated.

Keep Hydrated: Aim to drink plenty of fluids throughout the day, especially when consuming high-fiber foods like chia seeds. Water, herbal teas, and other hydrating beverages can support optimal digestive function.

The addition of chia seeds to a well-rounded diet provides a unique combination of fiber, hydration, and essential nutrients that work synergistically to promote healthy bowel movements. By understanding the connection between hydration and dietary choices like chia seeds, individuals can take proactive steps towards improving their digestive health and overcoming constipation. As we navigate the complexities of modern diets and lifestyles, prioritizing hydration and nutrition has never been more important for overall well-being.

Why Kids Need Plenty of Water

This chapter will explore the myriad reasons why kids need plenty of water, delving into its vital role in bodily functions, cognitive performance, physical activity, and long-term health benefits.

The Basics of Hydration

Water is a fundamental component of all living organisms, and children are no exception. Comprising approximately 70% of a child's body weight, water plays critical roles in various physiological processes. From maintaining body temperature to aiding digestion and nutrient absorption, hydration is integral to physical well-being. Children, due to their smaller bodies, have a higher turnover rate of fluids compared to adults, making adequate water intake even more crucial.

Body Temperature Regulation

One of the primary functions of water is to help regulate body temperature. Children are especially susceptible to overheating during play or physical activities. Sweating is the body's natural cooling mechanism, but sweat is composed primarily of water. If children don't replenish lost fluids, they risk dehydration, which can lead to a dangerous increase in body temperature. In extreme cases, overheating can lead to heat exhaustion or heatstroke, conditions that can have serious health consequences.

Supporting Digestion and Nutrition

Water is essential for effective digestion. It helps break down food so that the body can absorb nutrients effectively. Children are often habitual snackers, and a diet rich in fiber, such as fruits and vegetables, requires adequate water to assist in the proper breakdown of these foods. Furthermore, drinking water aids in the prevention of constipation, a common issue among kids who may not always prioritize eating enough fruits and vegetables.

Enhancing Cognitive Function

Hydration also significantly impacts cognitive performance. Studies have shown that even mild dehydration can impair attention, memory, and overall brain function in children. As children engage in academic activities or require concentration during school hours, having enough water can enhance their focus and learning capabilities. Hydration is particularly important in the classroom setting, where mental tasks demand a high level of concentration and cognitive processing.

The Role of Water in Physical Activity

Children are naturally active, participating in various games, sports, and physical activities. During vigorous exercise, the body loses water through sweat, and failing to replenish this fluid can lead to fatigue, reduced endurance, and decreased performance. Furthermore, dehydration can significantly affect a child's coordination and decision-making, putting them at a higher risk for accidents and injuries.

Teaching kids the importance of water intake before, during, and after physical activities not only helps them maintain their energy levels but also fosters a lifelong habit of hydration that extends beyond childhood.

Encouraging them to drink water before heading outside to play or to have a water bottle on hand during sports practice can ingrain this healthy habit.

Combatting Sugary Drinks

While water is often taken for granted, children are frequently drawn to sweetened beverages that promise a burst of flavor. Unfortunately, these drinks often contain high levels of sugar, which can lead to weight gain,

diabetes, and dental issues. Establishing water as the primary source of hydration can help combat these risks.

Parents and caregivers can play a pivotal role in shaping children's preferences by modeling water consumption as the norm. Providing water-rich foods, such as fruits and vegetables, and minimizing the availability of sugary alternatives can teach children that water is not just a necessity but a refreshing choice.

Creative Ways to Encourage Water Consumption

To ensure that children enjoy enough water daily, parents can get creative. Here are some tips to make hydration fun and engaging:

Infused Water: Adding slices of fruits like lemon, berries, or cucumber can enhance the flavor of water and make it more appealing.

Fun Containers: Using colorful, themed water bottles can encourage kids to drink more. Have them choose their favorite designs to foster a sense of ownership.

Hydration Reminders: Setting reminders or using

apps can help children track their water intake throughout the day.

Games and Challenges: Creating water-drinking challenges or games can turn hydration into a fun activity, encouraging friendly competition among siblings or friends.

Chia Seeds and Hydration

These tiny seeds, derived from the Salvia hispanica plant native to Central America, are celebrated not only for their rich nutrient profile but also for their remarkable ability to enhance hydration. This chapter delves into the intricate relationship between chia seeds and hydration, unraveling the science, practical applications, and potential benefits that come with incorporating this remarkable ingredient into our diets.

The Science Behind Chia Sees

Chia seeds are renowned for their high fiber content, boasting approximately 11 grams per ounce. This fiber is predominantly soluble, meaning that when chia seeds come into contact with liquid, they absorb water and swell to many times their original size. The result is a gel-like consistency that can help keep the body hydrated.

This unique characteristic of chia seeds stems from their high mucilage content, a substance that creates a gel when mixed with water. Mucilage not only aids in hydration by providing water retention but also contributes to a feeling of fullness, making it a valuable ally for those monitoring their weight.

Chia Seeds and Fluid Retention

When consumed, chia seeds can absorb up to 12 times their weight in water. This remarkable fluid-retaining ability means that when you include chia seeds in your diet, they can help bolster your body's hydration levels. This is particularly beneficial for individuals who engage in intense physical activity, as proper hydration is essential for optimal performance and recovery.

Athletes and fitness enthusiasts have increasingly turned to chia seeds as a natural alternative to electrolyte drinks. The combination of hydration and energy-boosting nutrients provides a dual benefit. When mixed into a smoothie or hydration drink, chia seeds can serve as a sustainable source of energy and hydration, supporting better performance and aiding in recovery.

How to Use Chia Seeds for Optimal Hydration

Incorporating chia seeds into your hydration regimen is both simple and versatile. Here are several ways to maximize their benefits:

Chia Seed Water: One of the most straightforward applications is to create a chia seed water. Mix one tablespoon of chia seeds in a glass of water and let them sit for 15-20 minutes until they form a gel. This concoction can be sipped throughout the day, providing a gentle hydration boost.

Smoothies: Adding chia seeds to smoothies enhances both texture and nutritional content. Combine your favorite fruits, greens, and a tablespoon of chia seeds for a hydrating and energizing drink.

Puddings: Chia seed pudding has gained popularity as

a healthy snack or breakfast option. Soak chia seeds in almond milk or coconut milk along with sweeteners and flavorings of choice. This silky pudding is not only delicious but also aids in hydration.

Baked Goods: Incorporating chia seeds into baked goods, such as muffins or energy bars, can yield both flavor and functional benefits. The added moisture from the chia seeds contributes to the overall hydration of the product.

Beyond Hydration: Nutritional Benefits of Chia Seeds

While the hydrating properties of chia seeds are a focal point, their nutritional profile offers a multitude of other health benefits. Packed with omega-3 fatty acids, protein, antioxidants, vitamins, and minerals, chia seeds contribute to heart health, digestive wellness, and overall vitality. The presence of calcium, magnesium, and phosphorus supports bone health, while fiber aids in digestion and may help control blood sugar levels.

As we continue to explore the nutritional landscape, chia seeds serve as a reminder of the interconnectedness of food, hydration, and well-being. Whether you're an athlete, a health enthusiast, or someone simply seeking to enhance their diet, chia seeds offer a simple yet effective way to nourish the body while maintaining optimal hydration levels. By embracing the magic of these tiny seeds, we unlock a world of health benefits that contribute to a vibrant and active lifestyle.

Chapter 7: Monitoring Your Child's Progress When Consuming Chia Seeds

Packed with omega-3 fatty acids, fiber, protein, and various essential minerals, chia seeds offer a multitude of health benefits. However, as with any dietary change, it is crucial to monitor how these tiny seeds affect your child's health and well-being.

In this chapter, we will explore several strategies for effectively tracking your child's progress when introducing chia seeds into their diet and understanding the potential benefits and challenges involved.

Understanding the Benefits of Chia Seeds

Before delving into tracking, it's important to recognize why you might consider chia seeds for your child. These seeds can contribute to:

Improved Digestion: Thanks to their high fiber content, chia seeds can help regulate your child's digestive system, preventing constipation and promoting gut health.

Increased Energy Levels: With their unique combination of protein and healthy fats, chia seeds can provide sustained energy throughout the day, which is useful for an active child.

Better Nutritional Profile: Chia seeds are rich in essential nutrients such as calcium, magnesium, and antioxidants, supporting overall health and development.

Healthy Weight Management: Their ability to absorb water and expand in the stomach can help your child feel fuller for longer, which could aid in weight management without feeling deprived.

Enhanced Brain Function: The omega-3 fatty acids found in chia seeds are essential for brain health, contributing to cognitive development and concentration during school activities.

Initial Guidelines for Starting

Before tracking your child's progress, it's essential to introduce chia seeds correctly. Start with small portions, such as half a teaspoon mixed into smoothies, yogurt, or oatmeal, and gradually increase to one tablespoon as your child becomes accustomed to the taste and texture. Always consult a pediatrician or nutritionist if you have any concerns or specific dietary needs for your child.

Strategies for Monitoring Progress

1. Keep a Food Diary

Maintaining a food diary can be incredibly helpful for tracking what your child eats, including chia seeds. Record details such as:

Portion Size: Note the amount of chia seeds consumed each day.

Meal Combinations: Document which recipes or dishes include chia seeds.

Overall Food Intake: Monitor other foods your child eats to get a broader picture of their diet.

This diary can help identify patterns related to chia seed consumption and your child's overall diet, making it easier to determine any changes in behavior or health.

2. Observe Physical Changes

Monitor any noteworthy physical changes in your child's health after introducing chia seeds:

Digestive Health: Have there been improvements in digestion, such as regular bowel movements? Or, conversely, are there signs of digestive discomfort?

Energy Levels: Observe if your child exhibits more consistent energy levels, particularly during school or playtime.

Skin and Hair Health: Keep an eye on any improvements in skin condition, hydration, or hair health.
3. Monitor Behavioral Changes

Diet can significantly affect mood and behavior, so it's important to note any changes in your child's temperament:

Mood Swings or Irritability: Have there been any noticeable changes, such as reduced irritability or increased happiness?

Cognitive Function: Pay attention to your child's focus and attention during tasks, both at home and in school settings.

Appetite: Monitor any shifts in your child's appetite, such as feeling fuller longer leading to less snacking.

4. Schedule Regular Check-Ins with Healthcare Professionals

Regular check-ups with your pediatrician or a nutritionist can help assess your child's health and the impact of chia seeds:

Nutritional Assessment: These professionals can evaluate if your child's diet, including chia seeds, meets their nutritional needs and whether adjustments are required.

Growth Monitoring: Regular check-ups include monitoring growth metrics such as height and weight to ensure your child is developing appropriately.

5. Engage Your Child in the Process

Involve your child in monitoring their own health and progress. This not only educates them about nutrition but also encourages responsibility and engagement with healthy eating habits. Ask your child about how they feel after meals, their energy levels throughout the day, and if they enjoy the taste of chia seeds.

Monitoring your child's progress when introducing chia seeds into their diet is vital to ensure they receive the benefits while minimizing any potential downsides. By keeping a detailed food diary, observing physical and behavioral changes, scheduling regular health check-ups, and engaging your child in discussions about their health, you can make informed decisions about their nutrition.

Keeping a Food Diary when consuming chia seeds

When coupled with the superfood chia seeds, known for their impressive nutritional profile and myriad health benefits, the practice of maintaining a food diary can become even more impactful. This chapter will explore the significance of a food diary, how to properly keep one while incorporating chia seeds into your diet, and the benefits that accompany this dual approach.

The Importance of a Food Diary

A food diary serves as a record of what you eat and drink throughout the day, allowing you to monitor your dietary habits, identify patterns, and hold yourself accountable. Research has shown that individuals who keep a food diary are more likely to lose weight and maintain healthy eating habits compared to those who do not. By documenting your food intake, you can:

Increase Awareness: Recording meals helps you become more conscious of what and how much you consume, making it easier to identify unhealthy patterns.

Understand Nutrients: A food diary allows you to analyze your nutrient intake, helping you ensure that you are meeting your dietary needs. This is especially beneficial when adding nutrient-dense foods like chia seeds into your meals.

Achieve Goals: Whether you're looking to lose weight, manage a health condition, or simply eat more mindfully, a food diary can help track progress and keep you motivated.

Incorporating Chia Seeds into Your Diet

Chia seeds, tiny powerhouses of nutrition, are packed with omega-3 fatty acids, fiber, protein, and a range of essential vitamins and minerals. Their versatility makes them easy to incorporate into various dishes—from smoothies and oatmeal to salads and baked goods.

Starting Your Chia Seed Journey

If you're new to chia seeds, introduce them gradually into your diet, noting different ways you consume them. Here are some suggestions for incorporating chia seeds and what to track in your food diary:

Breakfast: Add a tablespoon of chia seeds to your morning smoothie or yogurt. Record whether you notice any changes in your energy levels or satiety throughout the morning.

Snacks: Mix chia seeds into your favorite nut butter or blend them into a pudding. Document how these snacks affect your hunger and whether they keep you satisfied until your next meal.

Meals: Incorporate chia seeds into salads, soups, or baked goods. Keep track of what meals you enjoy the seeds in and how they enhance the overall taste and texture.

Hydration: Chia seeds absorb water, which can help with hydration. Monitor your fluid intake and note how well chia seeds help you maintain your hydration levels.

Keeping Your Diary

When keeping a food diary, consistency is key. Here's how to effectively document your chia seed consumption alongside your overall dietary intake:

Choose Your Format

Decide whether you would prefer a physical notebook, a dedicated food journaling app, or a simple spreadsheet. The choice depends on your comfort and accessibility.

Structure Your Entries Your food diary should include:

Date and Time: Note when you consume each meal or snack.

Food and Drink Items: Be specific about the foods

you're eating. For chia seeds, mention the quantity and how they were prepared.

Portion Sizes: Document the amounts you consume to get an idea of your intake.

Feelings and Reactions: Reflect on your mood before and after eating, any cravings, or satiety levels. This emotional context provides insight into your relationship with food.

Physical Reactions: Pay attention to any digestive changes or energy fluctuations, particularly as you introduce more chia seeds into your diet.

Weekly Reviews

Set aside time each week to review your entries. Look for trends in your mood and energy levels related to your chia seed consumption. Ask yourself questions like:

Did adding chia seeds help reduce my mid-morning snack cravings?

When did I feel most energized after meals incorporating chia seeds?

Are there certain meals where I enjoyed chia seeds more than others?

This practice not only reinforces positive habits but also provides a comprehensive view of how chia seeds influence your dietary experience.

Benefits of This Approach

By combining a food diary with the consumption of chia seeds, you may notice several positive outcomes:

Enhanced Nutritional Awareness: Regularly tracking

your meals helps elevate your understanding of nutrition and balance, particularly regarding the benefits of chia seeds.

Improved Digestive Health: The high fiber content in chia seeds may lead to improvements in digestion, which you can monitor through your diary.

Support for Healthy Habits: By being mindful of your food habits, you're more likely to make informed choices that align with your health goals.

Increased Motivation: Seeing your progress documented can be a powerful motivator, enhancing your commitment to healthy eating.

By documenting your journey, you not only gain insights into your eating habits but also cultivate a deeper appreciation for the foods that nourish your body. Embrace the experience, experiment with chia seeds in your meals, and watch as your food diary becomes a valuable ally on your path to improved health and well-being.

Identifying Improvement when consuming chia seeds

As more individuals integrate these tiny, nutrient-packed seeds into their diets, the quest for understanding their impacts on health becomes increasingly significant. This chapter aims to elucidate how to identify improvements in health and well-being when consuming chia seeds, highlighting key areas to observe and the science behind these observations.

1. Understanding Chia Seeds

Originating from the Salvia hispanica plant, chia seeds are an ancient food that has been cultivated for centuries by civilizations such as the Aztecs and Mayans. Packed with essential nutrients, chia seeds are rich in omega-3 fatty acids, fiber, protein, and a variety of vitamins and minerals. These small seeds have become popular not only for their nutritional composition but also for their versatility in recipes and ease of incorporation into various diets.

2. Tracking Physical Changes

One of the first areas to note improvements when incorporating chia seeds into your diet is your physical health. Numerous studies suggest that the consumption of chia seeds can contribute positively to several key areas:

Digestive Health: Thanks to their high fiber content, chia seeds can help improve digestion. When chia seeds are hydrated, they expand and form a gel-like substance, which can aid in regulating bowel movements. Individuals looking to track improvement should observe any changes in regularity and digestive comfort after consuming chia seeds daily.

Weight Management: Chia seeds may assist in weight control due to their ability to absorb large amounts of water and expand in the stomach, promoting a feeling of fullness. Monitoring appetite levels and changes in body weight over time can help assess their effectiveness as a satiating food source.

Hydration: As chia seeds absorb water, they can help

with hydration. Individuals engaging in physical activity or those living in hot climates may notice improvements in energy levels and overall hydration status when incorporating chia seeds into their post-workout nutrition.

3. Noting Mental and Emotional Well-being

The benefits of chia seeds extend beyond the physical realm. Numerous nutrients within chia seeds play crucial roles in mental and emotional health. Monitoring these areas can reveal significant improvements:

Omega-3 Fatty Acids and Mood: The omega-3 fatty acids present in chia seeds have been linked to brain health and mood regulation. Individuals may observe a reduction in symptoms of anxiety or depression, improved focus, or cognitive function after consistent chia seed consumption over time.

Energy Levels: Many users of chia seeds report increased vitality and diminished fatigue. Noting changes in energy levels during daily activities can be instrumental in understanding the impact of chia seeds on overall well-being.

4. Monitoring Skin and Appearance

Chia seeds contain antioxidants, which can help combat oxidative stress and support skin health. Improvements in skin conditions such as dryness, acne, or inflammation might be observed. Individuals should pay attention to:

Skin Hydration and Textures: Increased intake of chia seeds may lead to improved skin hydration and texture. Individuals can monitor their skin's appearance, noting any changes in smoothness or overall radiance.

Hair Health: Those attentive to hair health should consider any changes in shine, strength, or growth rate after incorporating chia seeds, which provide essential nutrients that support hair follicles.

5. Seeking Professional Guidance

While personal observations are invaluable, it may also be beneficial to seek professional guidance. Health professionals, such as nutritionists or dietitians, can provide tailored advice and support for identifying improvements based on individual health goals. They may recommend specific dietary adjustments, further investigation into food sensitivities, or detailed measurements such as blood tests to better assess the benefits of chia seeds on overall health.

6. A Holistic Approach to Health

While chia seeds offer numerous benefits, it's essential to adopt a holistic approach to health improvement. If one is consuming chia seeds as part of a balanced diet, alongside regular physical activity and adequate hydration, the positive effects can be magnified. Engaging in mindful eating practices and creating a supportive environment for health improvement will significantly enhance the experience and identification of positive changes.

Embracing chia seeds as a part of a balanced lifestyle can lead to profound transformations, driving home the truth in the adage that sometimes the smallest things can make the biggest difference. As the journey unfolds, each individual will find their unique narrative within the realm of chia seeds, celebrating the small victories that lead to a healthier, more vibrant life.

Chapter 8: Addressing Common Concerns When Including Chia Seeds in Children's Diets

These tiny, nutrient-rich seeds are packed with omega-3 fatty acids, fiber, protein, and various vitamins and minerals, making them an attractive addition to children's diets. However, as with any new food, concerns may arise. In this chapter, we will address common concerns that parents may have about including chia seeds in their children's meals, focusing on safety, allergies, digestion, and appropriate portion sizes.

Safety and Nutritional Benefits of Chia Seeds

Understanding Chia Seeds

Chia seeds (Salvia hispanica) have been consumed for centuries and were a staple food of the ancient Aztecs and Mayans. They are famous for their health benefits and are considered a superfood due to their impressive nutritional profile. With a high concentration of omega-3 fatty acids, chia seeds promote brain health, cardiovascular health, and overall well-being.

Safety Considerations

For most children, chia seeds can be safely included in their diets. They are often considered safe when consumed in appropriate amounts. However, it is crucial to consider a few factors:

Hydration: Chia seeds can absorb up to 10-12 times their weight in water. When consumed dry, they can swell and create a gel-like substance in the stomach, potentially causing discomfort or choking. To avoid this, always soak chia seeds in liquid (water, almond milk, or any preferred drink) before consuming them. This simple practice allows for easier digestion and mitigates any potential choking hazard.

Age Appropriateness: While chia seeds can be introduced into a child's diet around one year of age, it is essential to consult a pediatrician before doing so. Each child's development varies, and a healthcare professional can provide personalized guidance.

Allergic Reactions: As with any food, it is important to be aware of potential allergies. Although rare, cases of chia seed allergy have been reported. When introducing chia seeds, watch for signs of an allergic reaction, such as rash, itching, or gastrointestinal discomfort. If any concerning symptoms arise, discontinue use and consult a physician.

Addressing Digestive Issues

High Fiber Content

Chia seeds are an excellent source of dietary fiber; a single ounce provides approximately 11 grams. While fiber is vital for digestive health, introducing it too quickly into a child's diet can lead to gastrointestinal discomfort, such as bloating or constipation.

To avoid these complications, gradually increase fiber intake. Start with small amounts of soaked chia seeds (from 1 teaspoon to 1 tablespoon) and monitor how your child's digestive system responds. Be sure to encourage adequate fluid intake, as hydration can help the fiber do its job.

Incorporating Chia Seeds into Meals

There are various enjoyable ways to include chia seeds in children's meals:

Chia Puddings: Mixing chia seeds with milk or yogurt and letting them soak overnight creates a tasty, nutritious pudding that kids love. Enhance flavors with fruits, honey, or natural sweeteners.

Smoothies: Adding a tablespoon of soaked chia seeds to smoothies not only thickens the texture but also boosts nutritional value without altering the taste significantly.

Baked Goods: Chia seeds can be added to muffins, pancakes, or bread. They blend seamlessly into batter and provide added nutrition without being overly noticeable.

Toppings: Sprinkling chia seeds over oatmeal or yogurt can be an easy way to enhance breakfast. ## Recommended Serving Sizes

While chia seeds are packed with nutrients, moderation is key. Appropriate serving sizes for children vary by age and dietary preferences:

Ages 1-3: Start with 1 teaspoon of soaked chia seeds per day.

Ages 4-8: Increase to 1-2 tablespoons per day.

Ages 9 and up: Encourage a daily intake of 1-2 tablespoons, depending on individual dietary needs and preferences.

Parents should always consider the overall dietary context when including chia seeds. Balance is essential to ensure children receive a variety of nutrients from different food sources.

As with any new food, gradual introduction and

monitoring are crucial for ensuring a positive food experience. By incorporating chia seeds thoughtfully, parents can foster healthier eating habits that may last a lifetime.

Allergies and Intolerances in Children

This chapter aims to provide a comprehensive overview of allergies and intolerances in children, offering guidance to help families navigate the challenges they present.

Defining Allergies and Intolerances

Allergies are immune responses triggered by specific substances called allergens. When a child with an allergy ingests or comes into contact with an allergen, their immune system mistakenly identifies it as a threat, resulting in various reactions that can range from mild to severe. Common allergens for children include:

Peanuts

Tree nuts

Eggs

Milk

Wheat

Soy

Fish

Shellfish

Intolerances, on the other hand, generally do not

involve the immune system. Instead, these reactions occur when the body is unable to properly digest or metabolize specific foods, leading to gastrointestinal disturbances and discomfort. The most well-known food intolerance is lactose intolerance, which occurs when a child lacks the enzyme lactase needed to digest lactose, a sugar found in milk and dairy products.

Recognizing Symptoms

Identifying allergies and intolerances in children can be challenging, as symptoms can vary widely and may overlap. It's essential for parents and caregivers to be vigilant and aware of the signs that may indicate a problem.

Symptoms of Allergies

Skin Reactions: Hives, eczema, or swelling.

Respiratory Symptoms: Sneezing, nasal congestion, wheezing, or difficulty breathing.

Gastrointestinal Reactions: Nausea, vomiting, or diarrhea.

Anaphylaxis: A life-threatening reaction that requires immediate medical attention. Symptoms include difficulty breathing, swelling of the throat, a rapid drop in blood pressure, and loss of consciousness.

Symptoms of Intolerances

Gastrointestinal Distress: Bloating, gas, diarrhea, or constipation.

Headaches or Migraines

Fatigue or Lethargy: After consuming certain foods.

Skin Reactions: Though less common, some intolerances may also lead to rashes. ## Diagnosis

Diagnosing allergies and intolerances often requires a multi-faceted approach. Parents should maintain a detailed food diary to track their child's symptoms and potential triggers. Consulting with a pediatrician or an allergist can provide essential support in this process. Common diagnostic methods include:

Skin Prick Tests: A small amount of allergen is applied to the skin, and results are observed for reactions.

Blood Tests: These measure the immune system's response to specific allergens.

Elimination Diets: Removing potential allergens from the child's diet for a defined period and then gradually reintroducing them to identify triggers.

Management Strategies

Once a diagnosis has been made, managing a child's allergies or intolerances involves several key strategies: ### Allergen Avoidance

The cornerstone of living with food allergies or intolerances is strict avoidance of the offending substances. Parents should educate themselves about food labeling, ingredient lists, and cross-contamination risks in food preparation.

Nutritional Counseling

Children with food allergies or intolerances may struggle to obtain essential nutrients. Consulting with a registered dietitian can help ensure a balanced diet, providing alternatives and supplements when necessary.

Emergency Action Plans

For children at risk of severe allergic reactions, it is crucial to have an emergency action plan in place. This includes the use of emergency kits with antihistamines or an epinephrine auto-injector, as well as a clear plan communicated to schools, caregivers, and family members.

Education and Advocacy

It's vital to cultivate an ongoing dialogue about food allergies and intolerances. Educating children about their conditions empowers them to make informed choices as they grow older. Advocating for their needs in school settings, extracurricular activities, and social situations is equally important.

Allergies and intolerances present unique challenges that require careful management and understanding. By recognizing the differences between these conditions, identifying symptoms early, and implementing appropriate management strategies, parents can help their children lead healthy and fulfilling lives.

Potential Side Effects of Using Chia Seeds in Children's Diets

This chapter aims to explore the possible adverse effects of chia seeds on children and provide guidance for their safe consumption.

Understanding Chia Seeds

Before delving into the potential side effects, it is essential to understand what chia seeds are and their nutritional composition. Chia seeds are tiny black or white seeds that swell and form a gel-like substance when soaked in liquid. This characteristic not only enhances their texture when used in foods but also contributes to their high fiber content. For children, who require a balanced diet for healthy growth and development, the appeal of chia seeds lies in their potential to provide various nutrients.

Gastrointestinal Issues

One of the primary concerns when introducing chia seeds into a child's diet is the risk of gastrointestinal issues. Due to their high fiber content—approximately 11 grams per ounce—excessive consumption can lead to digestive discomfort. Children, especially, may experience symptoms such as bloating, gas, or diarrhea if they suddenly consume a large quantity of chia seeds.

Recommendations for Safe Consumption

To mitigate the risk of gastrointestinal distress, it is advisable to start with small amounts. A conservative approach might include:

Introducing chia seeds gradually into their diet, beginning with half a tablespoon.

Encouraging adequate hydration, as chia seeds absorb significant water. This is especially important when the seeds are consumed dry, as they can expand in the stomach and lead to discomfort.

Allergic Reactions

Although rare, some children may be allergic to chia seeds. Symptoms of an allergic reaction can range from mild (such as hives or rash) to severe (such as difficulty breathing or anaphylaxis). Parents should be vigilant when introducing chia seeds into their children's diets for the first time.

Allergy Testing

For children with a history of food allergies, it may be prudent to conduct an allergy test or consult with a pediatrician before introducing chia seeds. This can help ensure that children are not at risk of an adverse reaction.

Choking Hazard

Chia seeds can pose a choking hazard, especially for younger children. When dry, the seeds are small and hard, making them difficult for toddlers to swallow. When mixed with liquid, chia seeds expand and form a gel, which can also be a choking risk if not consumed properly.

Safety Tips

To minimize the choking risk:

Always serve chia seeds soaked in liquid, allowing them to expand before consumption.

Ensure supervision during meals if children are consuming foods containing chia seeds, particularly those under the age of four.

Nutritional Balance

While chia seeds can offer numerous health benefits, they should not dominate a child's diet. Overemphasis on any single food can lead to nutritional imbalances, which is particularly concerning in growing children. An overreliance on chia seeds may diminish the intake of other essential foods that provide varied nutrients necessary for healthy growth and development.

Holistic Dietary Approach

Parents should adopt a balanced approach, incorporating chia seeds as part of a varied diet that includes fruits, vegetables, whole grains, and proteins. This dietary diversity ensures children receive a wide range of vitamins and minerals crucial for their development.

By monitoring portion sizes, being attentive to allergies, ensuring proper preparation, and maintaining a balanced diet, parents can safely incorporate chia seeds into their children's meals. As with any dietary change, consultation with a healthcare professional or a registered dietitian can provide personalized guidance, ensuring that children's diets remain nutritious and enjoyable.

Chapter 9: Additional Natural Remedies for Constipation in Children

With an increasing number of parents seeking natural remedies and lifestyle adjustments to alleviate this common issue, it is essential to explore various alternatives. This chapter delves into additional natural remedies for constipation in children, highlighting dietary adjustments, hydration strategies, physical activities, and herbal aids that can help relieve discomfort and promote regular bowel movements.

1. Understanding Constipation

Before exploring natural remedies, it is fundamental to understand what constipation is. It is generally defined as having fewer than three bowel movements per week, with hard, dry, or difficult-to-pass stools. In children, constipation can result from various factors, including dietary habits, lack of physical activity, stress, and other medical conditions.

2. Dietary Adjustments

2.1 Fiber-Rich Foods

Increasing fiber intake is one of the most effective ways to relieve constipation. Try incorporating the following fiber-rich foods into your child's diet:

Fruits: Choose those high in fiber, such as pears, apples (with skin), bananas, strawberries, and prunes. These fruits not only provide fiber but also contain sorbitol, a natural sugar alcohol that can help soften stools.

Vegetables: Incorporate a variety of vegetables, especially leafy greens, carrots, broccoli, and peas. Raw vegetables can yield more fiber, so consider serving them in salads or as crudités.

Whole Grains: Replacing white bread and pasta with whole grain varieties can boost fiber intake. Oats, quinoa, and brown rice are also excellent options.

2.2 Probiotic Foods

Probiotics can help regulate the digestive system. Foods rich in probiotics include:

Yogurt: Look for those with live active cultures. Adding fruit to yogurt can make it more appealing to children.

Kefir: This fermented dairy drink is not only probiotic but can also be a delicious addition to smoothies.

Fermented Foods: Considering kid-friendly options

like sauerkraut or pickles can also enhance gut health.

2.3 Hydration

Staying hydrated is crucial for managing constipation. Encourage your child to drink plenty of fluids throughout the day, focusing on water and electrolyte-rich beverages.

Water: Aim for an adequate water intake suitable for your child's age and activity level.

Diluted Fruit Juices: Fruit juices, particularly prune, apple, or pear juice, can help move things along. Offer them in moderation, as too much juice can also act as a laxative.

Herbal Teas: Mild herbal teas like chamomile or peppermint can be soothing and hydrating, but always check with a pediatrician before introducing new herbal remedies.

3. Physical Activity

Promoting physical activity is a natural approach to help stimulate bowel movements. Simple activities can encourage digestion and regularity:

3.1 Active Play

Encourage unstructured playtime outdoors. Activities like running, jumping, biking, or even dancing can promote gastrointestinal health.

3.2 Regular Routine

Incorporate a routine that includes time for physical activity each day. Regular movement not only helps digestion but also improves overall physical and mental health.

3.3 Yoga and Stretching

Consider introducing gentle yoga poses designed to alleviate constipation, such as the child's pose, or simple stretches that engage the abdominal area.

4. Relaxation Techniques

Stress can be a significant contributor to constipation. Helping children manage anxiety and emotional disturbances is crucial for their overall health:

4.1 Mindfulness and Breathing

Teaching mindfulness exercises or deep breathing can help children relax. Engage in simple breathing exercises that emphasize slow, deep breaths, promoting relaxation.

4.2 Warm Baths

A warm bath can provide comfort and relaxation, making it easier for children to have bowel movements. Addition of gentle tummy massage while in the bath may enhance the relaxing effect.

5. Herbal Remedies

Before using any herbal remedy, consult with a pediatrician, especially since children may be more sensitive to herbs than adults. Some effective herbal options include:

5.1 Aloe Vera

Aloe vera juice in small quantities can act as a gentle laxative, but moderation is key. ### 5.2 Dandelion Tea

This herbal tea can help stimulate digestion and increase appetite. Ensure it is made mild and palatable for children.

5.3 Fennel Seed Tea

Fennel seeds can be brewed into a tea to aid digestion and reduce bloating. The taste is usually mildly sweet and pleasant.

6. When to Seek Medical Advice

While natural remedies can be effective for many children experiencing constipation, some situations warrant medical attention. If your child experiences the following, consult a healthcare professional:

Persistent constipation lasting more than two weeks.

Severe abdominal pain, cramping, or bloating.

Blood in stools or a family history of gastrointestinal issues.

Unexplained weight loss or changes in appetite.

While these remedies can be effective, it is essential for caregivers to be attentive to individual needs and consult healthcare providers for persistent issues. With these practical suggestions and a little patience, parents can help their children find comfort and relief from constipation, promoting not only digestive health but overall well-being.

Complementary Foods and Practices for Constipation in Children

As parents, caregivers, and healthcare providers strive to alleviate this condition, understanding the role of complementary foods and practices can be vital. This chapter will explore various complementary foods that can aid in promoting regular bowel movements and practices that can help alleviate constipation in children.

Understanding Constipation

Before delving into complementary foods and practices, it's essential to define constipation. Generally, constipation in children is characterized by infrequent bowel movements, hard or dry stools, and often discomfort during elimination. According to pediatric guidelines, a child is considered constipated if they have fewer than three bowel movements per week, or if they exhibit any symptoms such as straining, pain during bowel movements, or a feeling of incomplete evacuation.

Dietary Approaches ### High-Fiber Foods

One of the most effective dietary strategies to combat constipation is increasing fiber intake. Fiber adds bulk to stools and helps them move through the digestive tract more easily. Here are some high-fiber foods that can be incorporated into a child's diet:

Fruits: Encourage your child to eat whole fruits such as apples, pears, berries, prunes, and bananas. Prunes, in particular, are well-known for their natural laxative effect due to their high sorbitol content.

Vegetables: Integrating a variety of vegetables such as carrots, broccoli, sweet potatoes, and spinach into meals can significantly improve fiber intake.

Whole Grains: Opt for whole grain breads, cereals, and pasta instead of their refined counterparts. Foods like oatmeal and brown rice are excellent choices.

Legumes: Beans, lentils, and peas are not only rich in fiber but also provide protein and essential nutrients.

Nuts and Seeds: Almonds, chia seeds, and flaxseeds can be added to smoothies or yogurts for an added fiber boost.

Adequate Hydration

Alongside fiber, adequate hydration is crucial in maintaining healthy bowel movements. Children should be encouraged to drink plenty of fluids throughout the day. Water is the best option, but natural fruit juices (especially prune juice) can also support digestion. A good rule of thumb is to aim for at least 6 to 8 cups of fluids daily, adjusting for activity level and climate.

Meal Planning Strategies

Incorporating high-fiber foods into meals can be simple and enjoyable. Here are some strategies to help make meals not only fiber-rich but also appealing to children:

Smoothies: Blend fruits and leafy greens for a tasty and nutritious drink. You can add flaxseeds or chia seeds for extra fiber.

Baked Goods: Modify recipes for muffins or pancakes by substituting white flour with whole grain flour or incorporating oats.

Soups and Stews: Add beans and a variety of vegetables into soups and stews, fostering a hearty and fiber-rich dish.

Snacks: Choose fiber-rich snacks such as raw vegetables with hummus, popcorn, or yogurt topped with fruits and seeds.

Lifestyle Practices ### Physical Activity

Encouraging children to engage in regular physical activities can also stimulate the digestive system. Activities such as playing outside, riding bikes, or participating in sports can promote gastrointestinal motility and prevent constipation. Aim for at least 30 minutes of active play each day.

Establishing a Routine

Creating a regular bathroom routine can help children develop healthy bowel habits. Encourage them to set aside time after meals to sit on the toilet, as this aligns with the body's natural reflex to defecate. It's important to make this routine a non-stressful experience, as anxiety about using the toilet can exacerbate constipation.

Positive Reinforcement

For younger children, using positive reinforcement can be helpful. Praise them when they successfully use the toilet or maintain a healthy diet. Keeping the process light and encouraging can foster good habits without fear or stress.

When to Seek Professional Help

While many cases of childhood constipation can be managed at home with dietary and lifestyle changes, it's crucial to recognize when to seek professional help. If a child experiences severe pain, blood in their stool, or if constipation persists despite dietary modifications, consulting a pediatrician is essential. In some cases, a healthcare provider may recommend additional treatments such as over-the-counter laxatives or further evaluation.

By incorporating high-fiber foods, promoting regular exercise, and encouraging a positive toilet routine, parents and caregivers can significantly improve their child's digestive health and overall well-being.

Through these complementary foods and practices, constipation can often be alleviated, allowing children to thrive and engage joyfully in their daily lives.

Lifestyle Changes for Better Digestion for Constipation in Children

Addressing this condition often requires a comprehensive approach, starting with lifestyle modifications that can make a significant difference. This chapter explores practical lifestyle changes that can help improve digestion and alleviate constipation in children.

Understanding Constipation

Before delving into lifestyle changes, it's essential to understand what constipation is. In children, constipation is typically defined as having fewer than three bowel movements per week, and it may be accompanied by hard stools, discomfort, and straining during bowel movements. It is important to recognize that occasional constipation is common, but when it becomes chronic, it can impact a child's quality of life.

Dietary Adjustments #### 1. Increase Fiber Intake

A diet rich in fiber is fundamental in promoting healthy digestion and preventing constipation. Fiber helps to bulk up the stool, making it easier to pass. Encourage a diet that includes:

Fruits: Apples, pears, berries, and prunes are particularly effective.

Vegetables: Broccoli, carrots, spinach, and sweet potatoes can add essential fiber.

Whole grains: Opt for whole grain bread, brown rice, and oatmeal instead of refined grains. #### 2. Ensure Adequate Hydration

Water plays a crucial role in digestion. Encourage your child to drink plenty of fluids throughout the day, especially water. Proper hydration helps soften the stool and makes it easier to pass. A good rule of thumb is to aim for at least 6-8 cups of fluids daily, but this can vary based on age, activity level, and climate.

3. Limit Processed Foods

Many processed foods are low in fiber and high in unhealthy fats and sugars, which can exacerbate constipation. Try to limit consumption of:

Snack foods like chips and cookies

Fast food and takeout

Sugary cereals and soft drinks ### Establishing Healthy Habits #### 4. Regular Meal Times

Creating a consistent eating schedule encourages regular digestion. Try to seat your child for meals and snacks at the same times each day. This routine helps signal to their body that it's time to process food and can improve bowel regularity.

5. Promote Physical Activity

Regular physical activity is crucial for maintaining healthy digestion. Encourage your child to engage in age-appropriate exercises, such as:

Outdoor play (e.g., biking, running, playing tag)

Organized sports

Family walks or hikes

An active lifestyle can stimulate bowel movements and reduce the likelihood of constipation. #### 6. Encourage Healthy Bathroom Habits

Teach your child healthy toilet habits. Encourage them to use the restroom when they feel the urge to go, as delaying can lead to further issues. Creating a comfortable environment can help, so consider:

Allowing them privacy for longer durations

Keeping a stool nearby for foot support, which can help align the body for easier bowel movements ### Mindfulness and Relaxation

7. Reduce Stress

Stress and anxiety can affect gastrointestinal function. Encourage relaxation practices for your child, such as:

Mindful breathing exercises

Yoga or simple stretches

Engaging in hobbies that promote relaxation, like drawing or reading A calm state of mind can enhance digestive health.

8. Limit Screen Time

Excessive screen time can lead to a sedentary lifestyle, contributing to constipation. Implement daily limits on screen exposure, and encourage more active play instead. Designate times for screen use and promote family activities that involve physical movement.

Consult a Healthcare Professional

If lifestyle changes do not alleviate constipation, it's vital to consult a pediatric healthcare provider. They can provide guidance tailored to your child's specific needs, including further dietary suggestions or possible treatments. It's important to rule out underlying medical conditions that may contribute to chronic constipation.

By focusing on a nutritious diet, encouraging physical activity, promoting healthy bathroom habits, and maintaining emotional well-being, parents and caregivers can create a supportive environment for better digestion. A proactive approach can lead to improved gastrointestinal health, enhancing the overall quality of life for children and fostering healthy habits that can last a lifetime.

Chapter 10: Chia Seeds Beyond Constipation

Their nutritional benefits go far beyond promoting regular bowel movements. In this chapter, we will explore the multifaceted nature of chia seeds, delving into their rich nutritional profile, potential health benefits, and versatile uses that make them much more than just a digestive aid.

Nutritional Powerhouse

Chia seeds (*Salvia hispanica*) are small black or white seeds derived from a flowering plant native to Mexico and Guatemala. These tiny seeds are packed with nutrients: just two tablespoons (about 28 grams) contain approximately 140 calories, 4 grams of protein, 9 grams of fat (5 grams of which are omega-3 fatty acids), and 11 grams of dietary fiber. This unique combination of macronutrients and micronutrients makes chia seeds an exceptional addition to a balanced diet.

Omega-3 Fatty Acids

One of the standout features of chia seeds is their high content of omega-3 fatty acids, particularly alpha-linolenic acid (ALA). Omega-3s are known for their cardiovascular benefits, as they promote heart health by reducing inflammation, lowering blood pressure, and improving lipid profiles. As more people seek plant-based sources of these essential fats, chia seeds present a perfect alternative for vegans and vegetarians, helping to bridge the gap for those who do not consume fish or fish oil supplements.

Proteins and Fiber

In addition to omega-3s, chia seeds are an excellent source of plant-based protein, making them a valuable resource for vegetarian and vegan diets. They contain all nine essential amino acids, which are crucial for muscle repair, hormone production, and overall bodily function. The seeds are also high in fiber, which promotes not only digestive health but also increases satiety, which can be beneficial for weight management.

Micronutrients

Chia seeds are rich in essential minerals such as calcium, magnesium, phosphorus, and manganese. These minerals play important roles in bone health, energy production, and overall metabolic function. Incorporating chia seeds into your diet can help meet your daily nutritional needs, especially if you follow a diet that may be lacking in certain minerals.

Health Benefits Beyond Digestion

While chia seeds are widely recognized for their role in alleviating constipation, their health benefits encompass a broader spectrum and contribute to overall well-being.

Heart Health

As mentioned, the high ALA content in chia seeds is beneficial for heart health. Studies suggest that regular consumption of omega-3 fatty acids can help reduce triglycerides, lower blood pressure, and decrease the risk of heart disease. The soluble fiber in chia seeds also helps lower cholesterol levels, providing additional support for cardiovascular health.

Blood Sugar Regulation

Chia seeds may also help stabilize blood sugar levels due

to their high fiber content and unique gel-forming properties. When mixed with liquid, chia seeds absorb up to 12 times their weight in water, forming a gel- like consistency. This gel slows down the conversion of carbohydrates into sugar, resulting in a gradual release of glucose into the bloodstream, which is particularly beneficial for individuals managing diabetes or insulin resistance.

Weight Management

The combination of protein, fiber, and the gel-forming capacity of chia seeds contributes to a feeling of fullness and satiety. Adding chia seeds to meals can help curb hunger, reduce overall calorie intake, and support weight management efforts. These factors make chia seeds an excellent component of a balanced weight-loss diet.

Bone Health

With their rich mineral content, chia seeds can also play a significant role in maintaining bone health. They are an excellent non-dairy source of calcium, crucial for bone strength and density. Magnesium and phosphorus, found in significant amounts in chia seeds, also contribute to healthy bone mineralization.

Culinary Versatility

One of the best aspects of chia seeds is their versatility in the kitchen. They have a mild, nutty flavor and can be easily incorporated into a variety of dishes without altering the taste significantly. Whether you add them to smoothies, oatmeal, yogurt, or baked goods, chia seeds can effortlessly enhance the nutritional profile of any meal.

Creating Chia Pudding

Chia pudding has gained immense popularity as a healthy breakfast or snack option. To make it, simply mix chia seeds with your choice of milk or milk alternative, sweetener, and flavorings like vanilla or cocoa powder. Allow the mixture to sit for a few hours or overnight in the refrigerator. This creamy, nutritious pudding can be topped with fruits, nuts, and other toppings, creating a satisfying and wholesome treat.

As an Egg Substitute

For those exploring vegan cooking or reducing their egg intake, chia seeds can serve as a wonderful egg substitute. Mix one tablespoon of chia seeds with three tablespoons of water and let it sit for about 15 minutes, until it forms a gel-like consistency. This mixture can replace one egg in recipes, providing moisture and binding properties to baked goods.

While chia seeds have indeed carved out a niche as a remedy for constipation, their benefits extend far beyond digestive health. From supporting heart health to helping stabilize blood sugar levels, these tiny seeds are a powerhouse of nutrition. Their versatility in the kitchen means you can easily incorporate them into your daily routine, reaping the benefits of their rich nutrient profile.

Other Health Benefits of Chia Seeds for Kids

While they are well-known for their high omega-3 fatty acid content and fiber, chia seeds offer a plethora of other health benefits that make them an excellent addition to children's nutrition. This chapter explores these benefits, emphasizing their importance in supporting the growth and development of young bodies and minds.

Nutrient-Dense Powerhouse

Chia seeds are tiny nutritional powerhouses loaded with essential vitamins and minerals. Just a single ounce (about two tablespoons) provides approximately 18% of the daily recommended intake of calcium, which is crucial for children's bone development. Additionally, chia seeds are rich in magnesium, phosphorus, and manganese, all of which play vital roles in bone health and metabolic function.

Rich in Antioxidants

Another remarkable benefit of chia seeds is their high antioxidant content. Antioxidants help combat oxidative stress and inflammation in the body, which can reduce the risk of chronic diseases later in life. For children, whose bodies and immune systems are still developing, incorporating chia seeds into their diet can provide an essential defense against environmental toxins and stressors, supporting overall health and well-being.

Digestive Health

Digestive health is particularly important for children, as a healthy gut is vital for nutrient absorption and overall wellness. Chia seeds are an excellent source of dietary fiber, promoting healthy digestion and regular bowel movements. The soluble fiber in chia seeds can help create a gel-like substance in the stomach, which aids in slowing down digestion. This can ensure a steady release of energy and help children feel full longer, reducing the likelihood of unhealthy snacking.

Supports Healthy Growth

During childhood, growth spurts are common as kids develop at an incredible pace. Chia seeds can provide valuable nutrients that support this rapid growth. They contain a balanced ratio of protein, essential amino acids, and fatty acids, all of which are critical for proper growth and muscle development. Incorporating chia seeds into meals may help ensure that children receive adequate nutrition to support their burgeoning bodies.

Brain Health

The brain is one of the most vital organs, particularly during the formative years. Chia seeds are rich in omega-3 fatty acids, which are essential for brain health and cognitive function. Omega-3s have been linked to improved memory, focus, and overall brain performance. By introducing chia seeds into kids' diets, parents can provide a natural source of these necessary fatty acids, which could enhance their learning and developmental outcomes.

Natural Source of Energy

For active children, energy is crucial. Chia seeds offer a steady and sustainable energy source due to their unique combination of carbohydrates, protein, and healthy fats. Unlike sugary snacks that may lead to energy spikes followed by crashes, chia seeds can provide a more balanced and lasting energy release. This makes them an excellent addition to pre- or post-activity meals or snacks, helping children maintain their energy levels throughout their busy days. ## Supports Hydration

Chia seeds have a remarkable ability to absorb water—up to twelve times their weight. This property not only contributes to hydration but also makes them a perfect ingredient for smoothies, puddings, or drinks. Keeping kids well-hydrated is vital for their overall health, especially during hot weather or physical activity, and chia seeds can be a fun and tasty way to help achieve that goal.

Easy to Incorporate

One of the best aspects of chia seeds is their versatility. They can easily be incorporated into a variety of dishes without altering the taste. Parents can add them to smoothies, yogurt, oatmeal, baked goods, or sprinkle them on salads and soups. This ease of integration means that children can enjoy the numerous health benefits of chia seeds without fuss or significant changes to

Encouraging kids to try chia seeds and introducing them into meals can set the foundation for healthy eating habits that last a lifetime. As parents and caregivers, embracing the power of chia seeds may not only benefit children's health today, but also contribute to their well-being in the future. In the next chapter, we will explore fun and creative ways to serve chia seeds to kids, ensuring that they enjoy these superfoods while reaping all their benefits.

Long-term Dietary Inclusion of Chia Seeds for Children

One such food that has garnered attention for its impressive nutritional profile is chia seeds (Salvia hispanica). These tiny, nutrient-dense seeds are packed with omega-3 fatty acids, fiber, protein, vitamins, and minerals, making them a potential superfood for children. This chapter explores the long-term dietary inclusion of chia seeds for children, discussing their nutritional benefits, potential risks, practical ways to incorporate them into diets, and considerations for parents and caregivers.

Nutritional Profile of Chia Seeds

Chia seeds are often described as a "superfood" due to their nutritional density. They are an excellent source of:

Omega-3 Fatty Acids: Chia seeds are one of the richest plant-based sources of alpha-linolenic acid (ALA), an essential fatty acid critical for brain health and development. Omega-3s play a vital role in cognitive function, attention, and mood stabilization.

Dietary Fiber: High in both soluble and insoluble fiber, chia seeds support healthy digestion and can help prevent constipation—an issue many children face. The fiber content also promotes a feeling of fullness, which may help prevent overeating.

Proteins: Chia seeds provide all nine essential amino acids, making them a complete protein source, which is crucial for growing children during their development stages.

Vitamins and Minerals: Rich in calcium, magnesium, phosphorus, and zinc, chia seeds contribute to bone health and overall immunity, which is especially important for children.

Antioxidants: The antioxidants found in chia seeds can help protect children's cells from damage caused by free radicals, thus supporting overall health and wellness.

Benefits of Long-term Inclusion of Chia Seeds

Incorporating chia seeds into a child's daily diet might have several potential long-term benefits:

Cognitive Development: The omega-3 fatty acids found in chia seeds support brain health and development. Regular consumption might enhance cognitive function, memory retention, and overall academic performance.

Healthy Growth: The combination of protein, vitamins, and minerals found in chia seeds contributes to the healthy physical growth of children, helping to meet their nutritional requirements.

Digestive Health: The high fiber content supports a healthy gut, aiding in regular bowel movements and promoting a healthy microbiome, which can impact immune response and mood regulation.

Weight Management: The satiating properties of chia seeds may help prevent unhealthy snacking and contribute to maintaining a healthy weight during childhood and adolescence.

How to Incorporate Chia Seeds into Children's Diets

Given their versatility, chia seeds can be easily incorporated into a child's diet. Here are some practical ways to do so:

Chia Pudding: Mix chia seeds with milk (dairy or

plant-based) and sweetener or flavorings (such as vanilla or cocoa) and allow it to sit overnight. The seeds absorb the liquid, creating a pudding-like consistency that can be a delightful snack.

Smoothies: Add chia seeds to smoothies for an extra nutritional boost. They blend well and do not alter the flavor—a great way to include them without children noticing.

Baking: Incorporate chia seeds into pancake or muffin batter for added nutrition. They can also replace eggs in vegan recipes when mixed with water, helping to bind ingredients together.

Sprinkling: Sprinkle chia seeds on yogurt, oatmeal, or cereal as a crunchy topping. This not only enhances flavor but also increases the fiber and nutrient content of the meal.

Energy Bars: Make homemade energy bars containing chia seeds, oats, dried fruit, and nuts for a healthy snack that is both satisfying and nutritious.

Safety Considerations

While chia seeds are generally safe for children and can be included in their diets from a young age, there are important considerations to keep in mind:

Hydration: Chia seeds absorb a significant amount of liquid, expanding in size. Ensure children are adequately hydrated when consuming chia seeds to prevent digestive discomfort.

Allergies: Although rare, some individuals may have allergic reactions to chia seeds. Monitor for any adverse reactions when introducing them to the diet.

Choking Hazard: For younger children, it is advisable to soak chia seeds before consumption or serve them in dishes where they are mixed with other ingredients to minimize choking risks.

By incorporating these nutritious seeds in a variety of ways, parents and caregivers can support their children's growth, cognitive development, and overall health. As with any dietary addition, it is essential to consider individual dietary needs and preferences, ensuring a balanced and varied diet that promotes lifelong healthy eating habits. Embracing the versatility and health benefits of chia seeds can lead to a positive impact on children's nutritional intake and their journey toward healthy adulthood.

Conclusion

In conclusion, incorporating chia seeds into your child's diet can be a beneficial strategy to alleviate constipation and promote overall digestive health. These tiny seeds are packed with fiber, omega-3 fatty acids, and essential nutrients that can contribute not only to regular bowel movements but also to your child's overall well-being.

We've explored various ways to introduce chia seeds into daily meals—from smoothies and puddings to baked goods and snacks—making it easy and enjoyable for your kids to consume. Remember, the key to reaping the full benefits of chia seeds lies in proper hydration, so encouraging your child to drink plenty of water is equally important.

As with any dietary change, it's wise to introduce chia

seeds gradually and observe how your child's body responds. If you have any concerns about your child's digestive health, it's always best to consult with a healthcare professional.

By making chia seeds a fun and tasty part of your child's diet, you are taking an essential step toward promoting healthy digestion and fostering lifelong healthy eating habits. We hope this book has provided you with valuable insights and practical strategies to help your children thrive. Here's to happier tummies and healthier kids!

Biography

Alice Klayn is a renowned expert in the field of nutrition and digestive health, dedicated to transforming lives through the power of natural remedies and holistic wellness. With a background in nutritional science and over a decade of hands-on experience, Alice has become a trusted voice in the world of health and wellness.

Her passion for understanding the intricate workings of the human gut led her to specialize in addressing common yet often overlooked issues like constipation and overall digestive health.

As the author of her enlightening book, Alice dives deep into the secrets of gut health, offering readers a comprehensive guide to achieving optimal wellness. Her expertise in the benefits of chia seeds and other superfoods shines through, providing practical, science-backed advice that empowers readers to take control of their health.

Beyond her professional pursuits, Alice is an enthusiastic advocate for a balanced lifestyle. She enjoys experimenting with nutritious recipes, hiking in nature, and practicing yoga. Her personal journey with gut health challenges has fueled her mission to help others overcome similar obstacles and live their healthiest lives.

Alice Klayn's warm, approachable style and unwavering commitment to health make her an inspiring figure for anyone seeking to improve their well-being. Through her book, she invites you to embark on a transformative journey towards a healthier, happier you.

Read the QR code or click on the link to access your Bonuses!

Bonus 01: chia-seed-health-tracker-for-kids

qr.fm/0LyPk3

==================

Bonus 02: chia-seed-recipe-for-constipation-in-kids

qr.fm/eVuanO

==================

Bonus 03: chia-seeds-creative-meal-planning-for-kids

qr.fm/QWtO8w

Glossary: chia seeds for constipation kids

1. Chia Seeds:

Chia seeds are tiny black or white seeds derived from the Salvia hispanica plant, which is native to Mexico and Guatemala. They are rich in omega-3 fatty acids, fiber, protein, vitamins, and minerals, making them a nutritious addition to a balanced diet. Their unique ability to absorb water makes them particularly effective in promoting digestive health, especially for children suffering from constipation.

2. Constipation:

Constipation is a common digestive issue characterized by infrequent or difficult bowel movements. In children, it can cause discomfort, pain, and difficulty during toilet time. It is often caused by a lack of dietary fiber, insufficient fluid intake, sedentary lifestyle, or certain medications. Ensuring that kids have a varied and fiber-rich diet is critical in mitigating symptoms of constipation.

3. Dietary Fiber:

Dietary fiber is a type of carbohydrate that the body cannot digest. Fiber is essential for healthy digestion, as it adds bulk to the stool and facilitates its passage through the intestines. There are two types of dietary fiber: soluble fiber, which dissolves in water and can help soften stool, and insoluble fiber, which helps to move food through the digestive system. Chia seeds are an excellent source of both types of fiber.

4. Hydration:

Hydration refers to the process of maintaining adequate fluid levels in the body. Ensuring proper hydration is crucial in preventing constipation, as water helps soften stool and ease its passage through the intestines.

Chia seeds can absorb up to 10-12 times their weight in water, forming a gel-like substance that helps retain moisture in the stool.

5. Gelatinous Substance:

When chia seeds are mixed with liquid, they develop a gelatinous coating due to their soluble fiber content. This gelatinous substance can help bind water and create a bulkier stool, which can assist in easier elimination. In recipes for children, combining chia seeds with yogurt, smoothies, or oatmeal can ensure that they enjoy the benefits of this ingredient without noticing the change in texture.

6. Digestive Health:

Digestive health encompasses the proper functioning of the gastrointestinal system, which is vital for nutrient absorption and waste elimination. A diet rich in fiber, such as that which includes chia seeds, promotes a thriving digestive environment and can prevent issues like constipation in children.

7. Bowl Movement Regularity:

Regular bowel movements are a sign of a healthy digestive system. Children should typically have bowel movements anywhere from three times a day to three times a week. Consuming adequate fiber, such as that found in chia seeds, along with sufficient hydration, supports optimal bowel movement regularity.

8. Nutrient Density:

Nutrient density refers to the amount of essential nutrients in a food relative to its calorie content. Chia seeds are highly nutrient-dense, providing significant amounts of fiber, protein, and healthy fats without excessive calories. This quality makes them an excellent choice for kids, who require nutrient-rich foods for growth and development, especially during times when they might be experiencing digestive discomfort.

9. Incorporating Chia Seeds:

Incorporating chia seeds into a child's diet can be simple and enjoyable. They can be added to smoothies, oatmeal, yogurt, baked goods, or sprinkled on salads. The mild flavor of chia seeds makes them versatile and easy to include in a variety of meals and snacks.

10. Precautions:

While chia seeds can be beneficial, it is important to introduce them gradually into a child's diet, ensuring that they also consume plenty of water. Sudden increases in fiber without adequate hydration can lead to digestive discomfort.

www.ingramcontent.com/pod-product-compliance
Lightning Source LLC
Chambersburg PA
CBHW071223260726
48653CB00042B/1768